Love, Animals & Miracles

**Inspiring True Stories
Celebrating the Healing Bond**

DR. BERNIE S. SIEGEL

WITH CYNTHIA J. HURN

Foreword by Allen M. Schoen, DVM

New World Library
Novato, California

New World Library
14 Pamaron Way
Novato, California 94949

Text design by Tona Pearce Myers

Library of Congress Cataloging-in-Publication Data is available.

First printing, October 2015
ISBN 978-1-60868-334-5
Printed in Canada on 100% postconsumer-waste recycled paper

New World Library is proud to be a Gold Certified Environmentally Responsible Publisher. Publisher certification awarded by Green Press Initiative. www.greenpressinitiative.org

10   9   8   7   6   5   4   3   2   1

Contents

Thirteen: Grief and Forgiveness   233

Fourteen: Life Goes On   255

Foreword

There are many gateways to healing our emotional, psychological, and physical bodies. Bernie Siegel has studied, explored, experienced, and written about many of these approaches. Now, in *Love, Animals & Miracles*, he shares stories about what I feel are some of the greatest assistants in healing: our animal companions.

I have been a great admirer and friend of Bernie's for decades. As a matter of fact, my first book was titled *Love, Miracles, and Animal Healing*, a variation on the theme of his bestselling first book's title, *Love, Medicine & Miracles* (with his blessings, of course). In my book, I wrote about my healing journey and how animals can help us heal. Bernie and I would sometimes discuss our experiences about the healing power of animals. Occasionally he would contact me for advice about his animal companions. Most of the time, though, he already knew the answers he sought; my answers were simply additional confirmation of what he inherently knew.

Our mutual love of animals manifested itself in different ways. His led him to share his home with many animals as well as help his patients see and utilize the healing power of animals. My love of animals guided me to become a holistic integrative veterinarian, pioneering innovative, natural, nontoxic approaches to healing, from acupuncture to natural supplements to manual therapies. Our individual journeys intertwined again as we both recognized the healing power of the human-animal bond, though we arrived at that awareness via two different careers — two paths, two voices, yet one journey to the same destination, healing hearts, minds, and souls.

Our lives have paralleled each other's in many ways. When my mother was in an assisted-living facility near Bernie's home, whenever I visited her I heard all about Bernie's last visit to the home and how much he had touched the hearts of many who resided there through his talks to his resident support groups.

One of Bernie's life's themes has been about healing hearts. The metaphor of turning "swords into plowshares" may be adapted to turning "scalpels into love stories" with regard to Bernie's journey. During his personal spiritual journey, Bernie's goal was to be a healer. This first led him to become a renowned pediatric and general surgeon at Yale University. Through his conversations with his patients he began to realize that there was more to healing hearts than surgery. Perhaps before patients actually needed physical open-heart surgery, he could assist them in metaphysically opening their hearts by helping them heal from past traumas and wounds. Even after open-heart surgery, perhaps he could help them further open their hearts by guiding them through healing conversations and introspective personal explorations of self-help and healing. In his previous books, he shared conversations and stories illustrating that people can heal their hearts, and heal their cancer and afflictions of all kinds, much more quickly, if they get in touch with old mental and emotional programming that affects their immune systems and general health in numerous ways.

Bernie's stories in all his books are like lamps in the darkness, lighting a path of joy and hope for people dealing with the health challenges of cancer and other diseases. In this book, the stories shine a light on the healing power of the human-animal bond. They will bring a lightness of being to your day!

I love his stories about his family zoo. Sharing our homes with creatures great and small yields a deep intimacy. We learn so much from their individual behaviors and the beauty of how we communicate with one another every day. There are more multispecies households in the United States than ever before, and Bernie and Bobbie's home has certainly produced lots of uplifting stories from the far end of that spectrum.

Some of the stories in these pages, by our mutual friend Amelia Kinkade and many others, explore a more holistic and expansive view of our interconnectedness, transcending today's predominant, limited perspective of our relationship with animals. From trans-species communication, animal telepathy, and reincarnation to broader views of consciousness, Bernie dares to challenge current, limited belief systems. His stories offer viewpoints from critters ranging from dolphins and whales to tortoises and goats, as well as horses, dogs, and cats.

I pondered what I might share to adequately honor Bernie's writings while I meandered along the rocky, driftwood-covered Pacific Northwest beach below my island retreat cabin on one of the year's first warm spring days. The answers showered down on me along with rays of sunshine as I shared the beach with skinny-dipping hippies and playful sunbathing otters celebrating the glorious sun and warmth of spring. The loons were singing their song, eagles were soaring overhead savoring the shifting winds, purple starfish were sunning themselves just below the tide's surface, and schools of fish were swimming by. I spontaneously experienced the loving oneness that we all share beyond all of our minds' limitations and labels. I appreciated the continuous interconnectedness of all of us sharing that precious moment together. When one savors the healing powers of living together with all beings in peace and harmony, one realizes how vital it is to preserve natural environments that nurture our souls. Whether our families are limited to humans or expand out to our companion animals or even broader to all of nature, the magnificence of our interconnectedness unites us. Bernie's tales delight us with that awareness.

Savor all Bernie's stories and ponder how they help nourish your inner happiness, and then explore how you can go out and bring joy to others through them. We discover true happiness when we share happiness with others and watch them smile. That is why animals are so good at touching the deepest spaces in our hearts and can bypass our troubled thoughts and busy mind traffic. They can just ignite our inner light and infuse each cell with boundless, unconditional love, transcending our minds' endless doubts, worries, and concerns. May all these stories be teachers and healers.

Read, enjoy, and share Bernie's insights and stories, and be part of the change we all wish to see in the world! Thank you, Bernie, for offering all your amazing, heart-opening therapies and helping the world be a healthier, happier place!

— Allen M. Schoen, DVM, MS, PhD (hon.),
holistic integrative veterinarian and author of
The Compassionate Equestrian and *Kindred Spirits*,
www.drschoen.com

Introduction

Until he extends the circle of his compassion to all living things, man will not himself find peace.

— Albert Schweitzer

When our children were growing up, I would come home from the hospital after a long day of trying to save human lives, and if any of the animals in our house was injured or sick, the kids expected me to fix or cure their problems. That evening I might be sewing up a cat's wounds, bandaging a bird's wing, performing a cesarean section on a guinea pig, or operating on a turtle. I finally had to sit the kids down and explain that I couldn't save every creature's life and come home every night to more work after being a surgeon all day. Animals get sick and animals die.

I knew my kids were only reflecting what the animals teach us every day: that life is precious and the miracle of life stems from love. Our home was like a zoo, but one where all the animals were loved and considered family. Our kids saw animals as no less important than we were, even to the point that if I tried to kill an insect, such as a fly or a mosquito, they'd say, "Dad, let it out the door!"

I had been rescuing rainwashed worms for many decades and helping puddled insects out of trouble, all the while thinking I was neurotic. Then I came across an article by Albert Schweitzer. He said, if you're walking down the street after a rain, and you see an earthworm, put it back on the soil. When you find an insect in a puddle, give it a leaf to climb up on. Schweitzer's whole theme was reverence for life. That's what I realize we and the animals impregnated our children with. Throughout those influential years of character development, our kids were busy saving lives. Our home was an environment of love; and where love thrives, miracles happen.

Our children *expected* miracles, and they got them. When our dog Oscar developed a malignant melanoma, the vet said, "I've never seen a dog this sick recover. It would be better to euthanize him."

I didn't want to go home with a dead animal unless the kids agreed to this first. So I called home and told them what the vet recommended. I'll never forget their answer: "You don't put your patients to sleep. So you don't put Oscar to sleep."

I said to the vet, "I'm taking him home." Upon our return, Oscar was so weak he just lay on the floor. Over the next few days, if I had a meal, I shared it with Oscar, and I gave him vitamins. I would massage him and show him lots of love. In a few days he was sitting up; in a few more he was walking around the house; a week later I was letting him out with the other dogs — what's the point of staying indoors if you aren't dying anymore?

Oscar lived for three years with no sign of the cancer again. Anytime I met the vet, he'd shake his head in disbelief, repeating, "I never saw a dog that sick recover." It took me twenty years to realize it was the energy of love that did something to him, so that the cancer disappeared.

I know a doctor who said, "The best medicine is love." When someone asked him, "What if it doesn't work?" he replied, "Increase the dose." This is something animals do naturally. Unlike humans, who filter their love through intellect, animals give their friendship, compassion, and unconditional love wholeheartedly. If you are hurting, they don't leave you because they can't stand your suffering; they just love you more. These God-given qualities inspire humans to achieve greater heights of spiritual fulfillment.

Having a loving relationship with an animal is one of the most powerful factors in healing and maintaining well-being. Because of this, animals have been featured to some extent in all of my books. But this book is dedicated solely to the miracle of them and of their presence in our lives.

We've gathered stories from the Siegel household and from people who shared heartwarming and sometimes heartbreaking experiences, things that changed attitudes, enriched lives, and enlightened minds. When an animal touches a truth in us, this helps educate us and moves our consciousness into a higher plane. We have to write about it and talk about it, because we realize that it's now part of who we are.

In the following pages, animals are the teachers and the messengers. They are the doctors and the nurses. They are the miracle workers, the companions, and the sources and subjects of love. They are the guileless clowns who make us laugh. They are the extraordinary guides who pass through the curtain between life and death with their consciousness, showing us the true meaning of timeless eternity.

I invite you to settle into your favorite chair. Let the cat curl up in your lap, and keep one hand ready for stroking the dog when he nudges your arm. Then, join me on this journey as we explore the world of love, animals, and miracles.

1

The Siegel Zoo

She filled her own mouth with warm milk, put the wheat straw between her lips, and slanted the straw down to the mouth of the little racoon.... "This is the way you have to feed him, Sterling."

— Sterling North

The first thing you heard when you entered our house was chirping crickets, followed by an ever-varying mixture of sounds: squawks, purrs, chirrups, squeaks, barks, and so on, plus the talking, yelling, and laughter of kids and adults. When I tell people our house was a zoo, I'm not kidding.

Our circular street hems a rise of wooded acreage that is divided into several properties. On one side of our house, we fenced about thirty-eight hundred square feet for the animals and built a small barn at the end for the goats. In the mornings, when I would leave for the hospital, I'd let all the animals who preferred to be outdoors into this enclosure, where they'd stay until evening. Dogs, cats, goats, ducks, geese, skunks, squirrels, bunnies, and so on — all got along.

Inside the house, turtles lived in kiddie pools under artificial sunlight. I built platforms so they could climb out of the water, soak in the light, and go back in again whenever they wanted. Did the turtles get out of the pools now and again? Did I find turtle eggs in my shoes? Oh yes. Before I stepped into my shoes, I always tipped them up. If there was an egg — about an inch or so in diameter — it would roll to the heel. I'd take it out and put it in the incubator until it hatched.

Each of our five children had their own preferences for animals they raised. They educated themselves by attending lectures on the species they were caring for, and it was fascinating to hear them repeat what they'd learned.

Our son Stephen was the one interested in herpetology. We put a dead tree in his room, where, among snakes and other reptiles, he raised and bred Jackson's chameleons. These ate crickets, so he bred those too; and year-round, that end of the house sounded like summer. The chameleons wouldn't stay in Stephen's room. Sometimes you'd see them hanging from a painting in the hallway or in another unexpected place.

Among the guinea pigs and various other creatures Jeffrey raised were quail, for he was doing something with quail eggs. John had the keeshond dogs, named Oscar, Ike, and Nicky. Carolyn had the parakeet, Tweeter. And Keith, who was interested in pretty well everything, had tanks in his room for exotic turtles and frogs. While

Stephen's crickets brought summer to the household symphony, Keith's frogs made it sound like spring. My wife, Bobbie, and I had the cats — Miracle, Gabriel, Dickens, and Penny — and the smaller dogs. All these animals had cages or cardboard boxes where they slept at night, and the rest of the time they were free to wander through the house. We had creatures with fur, feathers, skin, and scales living in the house. I told visitors, "If you see a mouse running across the living room, don't scream. He's family." Sometimes it was hard to get babysitters. If they weren't comfortable with animals, they were in big trouble. We broke many zoning laws, but no neighbors reported us, nor did the police, because they knew it was done out of love for these creatures.

The largest animals we had were the goats. I'd be standing in the yard chatting with a neighbor, and suddenly, *wham!* There's a hoof on each of my shoulders. The goats used us as props to reach their favorite tree leaves. We also had ducks and geese in the yard, many of them hatched in the incubator. When the chicks hatched, the first beings they saw were our children, so the birds imprinted on them, thinking these human kids were their parents.

Every day the school bus would pick up our kids at the bottom of the drive. The ducks and geese would follow the kids, watch them get on the bus, and, when they were gone, waddle back to the yard. When the bus returned in the afternoon, the ducks and geese were already lined up, waiting by the road for their "parents" to get off the bus. Eventually we had too many waterfowl to keep them all at the house. My parents lived beside a lake, so we took the ducks over there and released them. Days later my mother called to say that every time a school bus turned up their road, the ducks deserted the lake and lined up for the bus, watching and waiting for their family to come home. Imagine that. It broke my heart, but the ducks needed a good place to live.

All our animals had names. We didn't talk about "the snake" or ask, "Where's the turtle?" We talked about Monty Python or asked, "Where's Paris?" A name might reflect something about the animal's personality or traits, as in the case of the racoons at our summer house on Cape Cod: Bobbie named them Raisin and Beggar. We wouldn't call a three-legged dog Tripod, focusing on its handicap. Instead we'd name it Hope or Luck. I could stand in the yard shouting, "Has anybody got Hope? I need Hope!" Or I might say, "Uh-oh, my Luck has run out."

One day I came home with *one more* rescued dog, and Bobbie said she didn't want any more creatures leaving "furphies" all over the furniture, which was what she called those little clumps they shed. Suddenly I knew — that's it! I handed her the dog and said, "His name is Furphy." Bobbie laughed.

"Okay," she said, "he can stay," and Furphy became family.

When we went on vacation, the animals came too. With five kids, the best solution to summer was a house on Cape Cod. We didn't bring the geese or ducks, but all the four-legged animals came, and we brought fencing to keep them safe. Everybody piled into the big suburban station wagon; the kids sat in the two front rows and the animals in the back. People would turn and gape as our car passed. You'd hear them say, "That's a goat!"

Before we left the house, we'd do a head count, which included the animals. Upon arrival at the Cape, everybody would go in and unpack, but there was always someone missing from the roll call. If you came in the house and thought, "Oops, there's a frog missing," you went back out to the car and looked until you found it hiding under the seat.

The kids also liked summer camp, where they were allowed to bring their animals. Our son Jeff brought his goat. The camp always had a pregnant cow, giving kids a chance to experience a delivery while they were there. One year the cow went into early labor on the day the camp opened, and I stepped in to help deliver the calf. The cow was lying down with all the kids crowded around, making noise and scaring her, and her labor kept stopping. I got the kids to be quiet and just watch.

I explained the process while petting the cow and reassuring her that all would be well, and then the calf finally appeared. I helped the calf out and taught the counselor what to do with the umbilical cord, the placenta, the mama cow, and her calf. It worked out very well, but I was sorry they didn't name the calf Bernie.

Living with a variety of animals, both at summer camp and at home, taught the kids respect for other living creatures, and it also blessed them with memories they still share and laugh about. Our daughter, Carolyn, had her bedroom next to Stephen's, making her vulnerable to the tricks brothers play on their sisters. Carolyn was happy to write down some of those memories for this book, and reading them made me laugh, bringing back so many wonderful memories. Allowing your children to grow up with animals is a gift that never stops teaching.

Growing Up the Siegel Way

CAROLYN SIEGEL MCGAHA

It was the rat snake who worried me the most; he had gone missing for several months. He had a reputation for getting away and showing up in the strangest of places. The first time he escaped, I took the cover off my old IBM typewriter to discover "Monty Python" curled on top, glaring at me with that intense snake stare. Of course I let out a whoop and holler, and my brothers thought it was hilarious. The next time Monty went missing, they started leaving rubber snakes outside my door. I'd wake up, open the door, step on the snake, and scream — great entertainment for them, but not for me!

I soon realized it was better not to react; I'd just pick up the rubber snake and fling it at my brother's door. One day I came out of my room, and there it was again. I reached down to pick up the fake snake…but it moved! I let out a blood-curdling scream and ran down the hall and into the yard, where my family was. I'd had such a scare I could hardly get the words out to answer the question "What on earth are you yelling about?" Finally, I screamed at Stephen, "Your snake — at my bedroom door!" The whole family ran into the house, and sure enough, there was Monty guarding my door. This time Stephen made the tank secure, making sure Monty Python didn't do his Houdini act again.

Another animal that used to go on walkabout was

the kinkajou, a nocturnal mammal from South America, sometimes called a honey bear. Kinkajous look like a cross between a monkey and a racoon; in fact, they come from the same family as racoons. Dad had rescued ours after someone abandoned it, and "Kinki" spent the evenings in a roomy cage downstairs. Once when I was about ten years old and my parents were away for a few days, we had a babysitter staying with us. I had noticed little powdered footprints all over my parent's bedroom, but I said nothing about it, even though it did seem odd, with them being away. Later that evening, company dropped in, and we gave them a grand tour of our big house with all the zoo animals. When I opened the door to the bathroom, talcum powder was all over the floor, and there was Kinki sitting on the toilet, just like a human. Days earlier Dad had put Kinki in diapers, but Kinki had scraped them off by dragging his butt on the ground. Maybe now Kinki was toilet training himself. It was the funniest thing we'd ever seen. We finally enticed our nocturnal friend back into his cage with a nice banana.

We were always rescuing animals and taking them in. Sometimes they'd been found wandering, or the local vet would call about an exotic animal that people could no longer cope with. We would observe Dad while he attended to their injuries, did emergency cesareans, or gave them mouth-to-mouth resuscitation. I loved growing up like that.

I had just got my driver's license when I saw an injured pigeon on the side of the road. I picked him up, put him in the back of my truck, and brought him straight home. Dad and I bandaged his leg and put him in the bathtub with food and water. We named him Louis.

It took several months to nurse Louis back to the state of health in which he could be safely set free. But when he was fully recovered and we brought him outside, Louis refused to leave! He flew into the tree, and for days he just stayed there. We put food out to make sure he was okay; then, after five or six days, Louis flew away, never to be seen again. It broke my heart, but knowing that we'd saved Louis and given him the freedom to make his own choice softened the blow.

Saving lives is a family tradition I carry on to this day. A few years ago, I purchased an Australian snake-necked turtle without knowing it had an ear infection. I came home and found it lying upside down in the turtle tank, not moving, not breathing. When I picked him up, his legs just dangled. I was determined to save him!

Holding him at face level, I began gently blowing air into his face, while pulling his front legs in and out, in and out, for over an hour, just like I had seen Dad do. The turtle took his first breath in a mighty gulp about twenty minutes into my work. Then water came out of his poor little nose. Finally, he came to and started moving around. As I drove him to the vet, such a beautiful feeling overwhelmed me. I had just saved a turtle's life!

Another time, Ginger, our toy poodle, choked on a piece of food that had fallen off the table. My husband said, "Ginger is having a seizure," but I realized from her purplish color and the lack of any sign of breathing that it wasn't a seizure. Inserting my hand down her throat, all the way to my wrist, I did the finger sweep, and pulled out a slice of onion that had become lodged in her windpipe. She immediately jumped up and started running around, so happy to be alive.

Several days ago we found a female snapping turtle that had been killed. Every year she used to make her journey from the pond across the road to my yard, where she'd lay her eggs. Sometimes she would be so exhausted after laying her eggs that we'd place her in a bucket, carry her back to the pond and release her. It was the least we could do.

I now felt it was my duty to save this turtle's offspring, so I called Dad to get his blessing for opening her up, and he replied with a yes. We managed to rescue all of her thirty-eight eggs. We placed them carefully into the soil where she used to lay, and we put wiring around the area to protect them from predators. We've since been eagerly awaiting the hatchlings.

Bernie's Comments

When your children are raised with animals and taught to be responsible for their care, you help your kids to become caring, gentle people. Our son Stephen recently wrote to me about his encounter with an animal in need of assistance.

Hi Dad,

I'm in Virginia for two weeks. I went for a walk yesterday near the woods and found this baby hatchling turtle all dried out and lying in the middle of the road. I picked him up and spent a half hour looking for a pond to let him go in. No idea how he got in the middle of the highway to begin with. He must have been really lost and didn't want to ask directions (that's how I knew it was a male turtle).

Stephen went to law school and became an FBI agent. It really shook me at the commencement ceremony when I learned that agents' work requires them not only to carry a gun but also to be prepared to use it. So when I read his email I was thinking, "Here's a guy with a gun who goes out of his way and spends half an hour just to help a turtle." And I was so proud of him. No matter what may happen to him while in the line of duty, he had been impregnated with the understanding that we are here to save lives, and he carries that with him wherever he goes. He sees the funny side of things too. Laughter is a great healer when we're sick, and it strengthens our immune system during times of stress.

Animals often inspire us to create. When I write poetry, it helps me to make sense of the world or to have a good laugh at myself, especially when it includes the animals, as in the following poem.

What Is So Important I Can't Sleep

I need to get out of bed
And then I will write my book
And then I will enlighten the world
And then I arise
And then I uncover the rabbit cage
And then I open the cage
And then I rub her back
And then I feed her
And then I clean the cage
And then I clean the fish pond
And then I clean the kitty litter
And then I let our cats out
And then I fill the bird feeders
And then I walk our dog
And then I jog to Jeff's house
And then I pet his lonesome cat
And then I use his exercise equipment
And then I feed his dogs

And then I check on his chickens
And then I feed his ducks
And then I go home
And then I eat breakfast with my wife and pets
And then I decide what my life is truly about
And to write the book tomorrow

2

Becoming Family

He needed the companionship of a family member. Someone who was there for him, who had proven time and time again her devotion to him. He slept as a child curled up in her [elephant] trunk. His tears were known only to her.

— Ralph Helfer

The main building block of any society has always been family, followed by community. Ancient books, such as the Bible, teach about a spiritual family, one drawn "of all nations, and kindreds, and people, and tongues" (Revelation 7:9). The defining characteristic of a spiritual family is *love for one another*.

Consider a line in one of Robert Frost's poems: "Home is a place where, when you have to go there, they have to take you in." Think how secure you feel if you know that no matter what happens in your life, your family will let you in. That's powerful.

One day while we were at a family event, I was looking at my mother, when it suddenly hit me that every single person in the room was alive because of her; they came from her. It struck me then how incredibly important each and every being is. Without them, so much would never exist — would never happen. Whether it's Adam and Eve or your mother and father, we're talking about the beginning of life: it just expands and goes on.

When we help another living thing, we are immortalizing ourselves, kids or no kids. We are giving birth to spiritual family. Lloyd Biggle Jr. said to "guard the life of another creature as you would your own, because it is your own." Animals accept you as family; when you feel their love — the sharing, the forgiving — you know they're attached to you, and your life is not empty.

When I traveled while giving lectures, it was lonely. Eventually my wife, Bobbie, traveled with me, so I didn't leave home behind; home came with me. Bobbie was usually the one at our house who got up in the morning and fed everybody, and the cats took it upon themselves to wake her up. They would climb onto her chest and do that kneading motion with their paws. One morning we were in our hotel room. We had to go and give a lecture, but Bobbie was fast asleep. I went to her with my fingers curled, mimicking a cat's paws, and started kneading her chest. She woke up thinking, "Ahh, the sweet cats." But when she opened her eyes, here's this guy leaning over her, and she let out such a shriek. What a fun way to get her up. It was so funny I wrote a poem about it, called "Awaken, My Love."

AWAKEN, MY LOVE

It's time to get up
but we are not at home
no living alarm clock
no cats to purr
pounce on her chest
awaken her with a cold nose on her chin
I love her
so I do my best
I pounce on her chest
purr loudly
and put my cold nose on her chin
it works
she awakens
with a smile
to my love

When Bobbie couldn't travel with me, I started bringing our dog Furphy, and once again home came with me. That's what they do. The bed is warm and cozy; you can relax and sleep; your whole day is different because you didn't go to sleep and wake up lonely. We know that loneliness affects the genes that control immune function, making you vulnerable to illness and other problems.

Animals let you know you are loved, and they make

you laugh when you need it. All those things help us stay healthy and live longer. If there is a void in your life, an emptiness that you cannot fill, go and find an animal. Make them your family. The void will disappear, and love will take its place.

The following stories involve animals whose presence contributed to the well-being of their human family, sometimes to the point of saving their lives.

Black Velvet

Jeanna Barrett

The runt of the litter was a tiny scrap of black velvet already showing a feistiness that belied her fragility at the beginning. She was unable to leave her mother when the other kittens were adopted, and I had to wait an extra two weeks before collecting her from the farm in the English countryside. I brought her home in a cardboard box. She cost me five pounds sterling.

I wasn't really a cat person, preferring the various breeds of dogs I had been brought up with. Working as a flight attendant, however, meant being away from home a great deal, so having a dog wasn't an option. I needed a companion, and that is how Tai-Lu came into my life and stayed for the next eighteen years.

For the first six months she drove me mad — hanging off the curtains, scratching the furniture, and bringing me an array of unwanted presents. Frogs, dragonflies, baby birds, and other half-dead creatures were regularly deposited on the kitchen floor. While hunting was her pride and pleasure, she resolutely failed in her bounden duty of catching either the mice that holed up behind the fridge or — my nemesis — large, hairy spiders! Tai-Lu loved to hide in drawers and other obscure places, including my ready-packed suitcase. On one occasion she emerged from under the clothes just as I was lowering the lid.

Many a time I wondered what on earth had I done, adopting this kitten, but a day came when I realized just how much she meant to me. I bent down to her and said, "I *do* love you." Tai-Lu gave a loud "Mew!" and gently reached out her paw to touch my hand. That was the start of the most wonderful bond between us.

My neighbor always knew when I was due home from a flight, because Tai-Lu would appear, sometimes up to two hours before my arrival, and sit on the pavement outside my house. As soon as I opened the car door she would jump onto my lap, purring loudly. Later, I moved to a Somerset village far from the city, but I was still working out of Heathrow. Exhausted after a long-haul flight, I would then be faced with a two-and-a-half-hour drive home. When I got there Tai-Lu would be sleeping in her favorite place, a sunny spot under the beautiful *Ginkgo biloba* tree in the back garden. I'd tap on the kitchen window, and she'd wake, rush across the grass, and tumble through the cat flap, winding herself around my legs, mewing with pleasure at my homecoming. I'd scoop her up and hold her close while she reached her paws around my neck and nuzzled my face. The affection she always showed me was extraordinary — and deeply comforting.

Looking back on our time together, I truly believe my black velvet companion was (and is) one of my guardian angels. Once when I was getting out of bed, I collapsed on the floor in absolute agony, completely helpless to get up, not knowing (until later) that I had just torn three discs in my spine. Somehow I managed to reach the phone. As I lay on my stomach waiting for help to come, Tai-Lu knew exactly what I needed. She climbed gently onto my lower back and curled up, giving out the most amazing healing warmth. She stayed put until my neighbor let the doctor in; and even then, she refused to move, hissing furiously as she tried to protect me from the longed-for injection of morphine.

Another night she stopped me from taking my own life when I was drunk and severely clinically depressed. Tai-Lu appeared from nowhere and sat with me, pressing herself as close as she could to my body. I just couldn't do it; I loved her too much to leave her.

I've been told that our animals are sent to us as healers, teachers, or companions. Tai-Lu was a true healer, a loyal and comforting presence throughout all my heartaches, doubts, and loneliness. There were times when I don't know what I would have done without her. She was the one constant in my life during long years of living out of a suitcase — the only one always there to come home to.

In her last years Tai-Lu was plagued with illness, and I was glad to retire from the airlines in order to look after her better. A few weeks before her eighteenth birthday, I knew the end was close. She had stopped eating and was uncomfortable. For three days I fed her water from a teaspoon and changed her soiled bedding, since she could no longer stand up. I couldn't face losing her and loathed the thought of committing her to a vet. In the end I just prayed hard that she would go to sleep and be at peace. The next morning I went downstairs and found my sweet Tai-Lu had died in the night. I knelt by her bed and whispered, "Dearest Tai-Lu, thank you for sharing one of your lives with me. I will see you on Rainbow Bridge, little one."

Bird Bravery

BARB BLAND

Chilled by the morning fog, I tucked the newspaper under my arm and scuttled back to the house, when a terrible sight stopped me in my tracks. There on the cold concrete beneath the kitchen window lay three naked barn swallow chicks surrounded by crumbled bits of dried gray mud, their fallen nest.

Barn swallows had always nested under our front eaves. "Lord and Lady Chatterley" often perched on the overhead wires chortling to each other as we went about our front-yard tasks. One of their most endearing habits involved sunning themselves atop the doghouse or the electricity meter. The birds would gasp and pant in the heat as they changed position, like bathing beauties rotating for an even tan. Their trust in us was clear, for they allowed us to stand almost close enough to touch them.

But now there was no sign of the parents, and the unmoving chicks looked dead. I gently touched one of the baby birds. The blue bulges of its unopened eyes highlighted the iciness of its skin. Carefully checking the others, I found that none of them were rigid. On closer inspection, a faint pulse in their blood vessels was visible through the almost transparent, pale pink skin.

Nestling three limp bodies in the palm of my hand, I went inside, turned on the heater, and stood next to the wall vent, which instantly poured out warmth. Cupping my hands over the hot air, I held the helpless birds skin to skin, the most efficient transfer of heat.

My husband returned from walking the dog, so I recruited his big warm hands to hold the chicks over the heater while I gathered things I'd need in order to care for them. I'll never forget his delighted smile when, after a few minutes, they began to wobble and squirm in his hands.

After lining an empty margarine tub loosely with tissues, I placed it into a small cardboard box for more stability. I then built a tower of plates on the stovetop and placed the cardboard box on the top plate, six inches below the range light. Settling the chicks into the tissue nest, I laid more tissue loosely over them, protecting the chicks' tender skin from the bulb's direct heat.

The chicks now began screaming for food. It had probably been hours since they'd eaten, perhaps not since the previous night. The parents had generously supplied them with fresh flies and other small insects, but I was no swallow. What could I possibly do?

Opening a jar of mashed meat baby food, I scooped out a tiny amount with the flat end of a wooden toothpick. I gently pinched one chick's tiny cartilage beak between my fingers, causing its mouth to open wide; then I touched the inside corner of its mouth with the food, causing it to swallow reflexively. The feeding sequence from chick A to B to C took a while, but eventually they filled up enough to contentedly nod off.

I glanced at the time — 8:10 AM. It had been 6:30

when I went to get the paper. I decided I'd better have a look for the parents. Fog still sifted between the houses, and no birds were in sight. Returning to the kitchen, I made breakfast for us and stuffed another round of food into the chicks' gaping, hungry mouths, fully aware that I couldn't save them; they needed their parents' care. Somehow, I'd have to get a nest back under the eaves. Birds relate to one another by sound, not by smell as mammals do. The parents might not reject their young in response to my touching them, but would they resume their care?

I stretched sturdy rubber bands around a larger margarine tub, then climbed a stepladder and drove three nails into the wall. I wove the rubber bands around the nails and checked to see if they would hold. The construction seemed to work, but the shiny yellow plastic was a far cry from the matte gray mud of a real swallow's nest.

Fluttering wings sounded behind me. One of the parents was hovering in seeming disbelief that its human had destroyed its nest. The other parent perched on the overhead wires. Was this a betrayal of trust? Frightened, they flew away. I climbed down, disheartened and worried.

Nine-thirty. I fed the chicks again. Then I slipped the chicks' margarine tub into the larger one on the wall and went inside to watch. Seated on the kitchen floor with my eyes glued to the nest, I waited and prayed.

Ten o'clock. Ten-thirty. Should I feed the babies?

While I was making the effort to stand up, something flickered in the window. Sunlight reflecting from the plastic tub grew brighter and then faded. I went outside to find that the fog was lifting and clouds behind it were breaking up. Aha! Lord and Lady Chatterley perched nearby, studying the nest.

Back I went to the hard floor, this time filled with hope.

Eleven o'clock. Those chicks needed to eat.

As I contemplated making a move, the miracle breakthrough finally happened. One of the parents overcame its fear, flew to the margarine tub, perched on the edge, and briefly examined the chicks before flying away. The other parent then arrived with an insect in its beak and offered it to the hungry chicks.

Lord and Lady Chatterley proceeded to raise their brood. Over the next few weeks, the nestlings' eyes opened and feathers grew. The youngsters fledged, attended flight school, and are now raising families of their own. Our willingness to try, and the birds' bravery in overcoming their fear of a strange nest, saved the lives of their chicks and of the many generations to come.

The Long Wait

JANICE PETERS

Mowgli arrived at Best Friends Animal Society in Utah after being rejected by two shelters. On my day for volunteering, I saw the eight-month-old malamute sitting off by himself, and I walked over to the fence to talk to him. When those mahogany eyes looked deep into my heart and touched my soul, I fell in love.

His caregiver said he was unapproachable. But when we entered the run, I knelt down and held out my hand; Mowgli walked up and let me touch his nose. I was ready to take him home that day, but he wasn't cleared for adoption yet. As soon as he was cleared, my offer was rejected because of his shyness and the two alpha huskies I already had at home.

Eight years later, both huskies were gone, and Mowgli was still at Best Friends. I brought Sami, my border collie, to meet him. After all that time, Mowgli let me approach him once again! He and Sami got along well, so Mowgli came home at last.

Mo was still extremely shy, and he feared touch. He also disliked closed rooms. But he seemed comfortable with us; since my house has a circular floor plan, he could always get to the dog door and the yard. He chose a sleeping spot in the hallway outside my bedroom, where he could see Sami and me and still have a direct path to the exit.

To encourage his trust, I held Mo's food dish while he ate. I didn't touch him, but just spoke quietly and praised him when he was finished. He was always wonderfully gentle, never grabbing at treats but taking them with his lips. Quick movements startled and disturbed him, so I learned to slow down when walking from room to room and to gesture in the direction I was headed.

Mo learned by watching. Observing the nightly strokes and cuddles I gave Sami, he began to stand close to us and let me scratch just his ears and nose. After several months my patience paid off; he put his head in my lap and, for the first time, I petted him properly.

Mowgli was extremely sensitive to my moods and voice. I learned to be calmer and to speak quietly. On the occasions when I raised my voice to imply he'd done something wrong, that volume was all the punishment he needed — the lesson was learned.

For all his shyness, Mo had a great sense of humor. He loved his squeaky toys, carried them around, slept with them, and amused himself with them. A neighbor told me that whenever I'd leave the house, Mowgli would take his toys out on the deck, arrange them in a tableau, and then rearrange them. I'd come home to these displays, which always made me laugh.

It took a long time to get Mo into my van after his twelve-hour trip home from Best Friends. He did *not* want to be enclosed like that again. It was almost a year before he finally decided to chance it. I immediately took him to the beach…the first time he ever saw the ocean. After that, car rides were a much-enjoyed activity.

While shy with people, Mo was wonderful with other dogs. Big as he was, he remained completely gentle with dogs we'd encounter, even if they acted aggressively toward him. It was magical to watch his calmness calm them down. Mowgli never acted upset about anything. He'd observe, and you could see him thinking things through. A friend called him a lone wolf, and that fit. Unlike any other dog I've had, Mo maintained an aloofness that suggested he wasn't completely of this world, even though he enjoyed the experiences it offered.

Mowgli was nine when I adopted him, and he weighed 115 pounds. I had known I wouldn't have him for too many years, but only eighteen months later he developed bone cancer. The most difficult thing for any pet owner is deciding if it's better to help them go than it is to help them stay. Again I took my cue from Mo: as long as he wanted to go for walks, sleep on the deck, and play with his toys, I kept him comfortable. One day we went for a short walk and then drove next to the beach. He always enjoyed looking at the ocean, but this time he was especially attentive. I thought, "He knows it's the last time he'll see this."

We came home, had a long cuddle session, then sat on the deck and watched a beautiful sunset...a peaceful last evening. When the light caught his eyes, turning them bright turquoise-green, he truly looked like a wolf — ready to embrace his spirit.

The next day, before the vet arrived, Mowgli and I settled on the deck with Sami. I told Mo how grateful I was that he had waited for me and came home with me. When the vet finally came, I held Mo's face cradled on my chest, stroking his head and back. Completely calm, he kept his eyes on me the whole time until he went under, with me whispering, "I love you, Mo," in his ear.

The last thing Mowgli taught me is that love has no time limits. I loved him for eight years from afar and eighteen months while we were together. It's been six years since he died, but his place is still here — in my heart — forever.

My Boy Rusty

Doreen Semmens

≈≈

He was just a little guy at nine weeks of age, the color of champagne, with big paws and a wide forehead that made me believe he would be very intelligent. Little did I know just how intelligent he'd be! His mother, a white Maltese terrier, and his father, a black poodle, had created between them a genuine Maltipoo.

The puppy was to be my Christmas present from my husband, but we couldn't take him home for another four weeks, not until he was old enough to leave his mother. When we finally did collect him, I felt so sorry for her. How awful to have your baby taken away. We named the puppy Rusty.

I have to admit that, at seventy-two years of age, I had forgotten how much hard work puppies could be, but we survived the holes dug in the lawn, the destruction of my husband's books that were chewed up, the requests and demands to play the moment we sat down to watch the news, and the constant outings necessary to get him house-trained.

Rusty soon became an equal member of the family; everywhere we went, Rusty went too. He quickly grew wise to the fact that if he wagged his tail and smiled at people (yes, a full, toothy grin), they would pat him and tell him what a cute little guy he was. I'm not going to say that he didn't have naughty moments, like the time he blatantly stole a sandwich from a friend's hand when we were out on a picnic and then devoured it, leaving my husband and me with no option but to share what was left of our lunch. But the disarming smile always won him everyone's forgiveness.

We made many new friends because of Rusty. As the years wore on and our hearing got worse, Rusty became our ears, barking to let us know if the doorbell or telephone rang.

My husband had to spend the last six months of his life in a care facility. Every day Rusty and I would visit him, and we were allowed to attend the various social activities as a family. Rusty brought a smile to so many faces. The residents looked forward to seeing his comical little face and stroking his soft furry coat. He would look back at them with such gratitude and joy, it made their day. One dose of Rusty therapy was good for the whole day.

Rusty doesn't hear the phone ring anymore, or the doorbell. He's going on sixteen years, and he's wondering where his dad is. My husband passed away on Christmas Day, but Rusty never got the message, or maybe he just wasn't ready to receive it. He still stands at the top of the stairs, waiting for the door to open and his dad to come home. I'm not ready to lose Rusty yet, but I know I have to prepare myself, for one day that door will open and my sweet boy Rusty will be with his dad again.

Bernie's Comments

In "Black Velvet," when Jeanna said to her cat, "I *do* love you," her cat got the message; she knew what Jeanna felt, the same way Tai-Lu understood what was happening during the times Jeanna was hurting, physically or mentally, and the cat tried to save her.

I heard of one couple who claimed their cat always knew when their daughter was returning from work. A researcher rigged up a web cam aimed at the window where the cat awaited the daughter's arrival. The daughter came home at different times, using a variety of transportation methods to eliminate the possibility that the cat simply recognized the sound of her car. The daughter would show up an hour early, an hour late. Every single time, with only two exceptions, the cat appeared at the window minutes before she arrived. The two times he didn't, the neighbor's cat was in heat. Apparently sex trumped loyalty.

Dying at night — as Jeanna's cat did — is no coincidence. Ask any nurse: most people who die in a hospital do so at night. It's peaceful, with no distractions, no family to feel guilty about leaving, and no doctor to stop you. You also don't want your family to feel distressed. Dying kids do that too, trying to make it easier on the parents who remain by their side around the clock. Parents will go down to the cafeteria and come back to find their child has died. They feel awful that they weren't there, but I tell them, "No, your child was doing that for you."

In Barb's story, "Bird Bravery," the humans acted with the knowledge that all life is connected; regardless of species, we are of the same family. The bird parents understood what the human "godparents" had done for their babies. Like my mother, whose life made many others' possible, this human couple became the givers of life.

In Janice's story, "The Long Wait," Mowgli is like a Zen master, quiet and at peace. It's hard — when animals have cancer or some other devastating condition — to choose for them. When I make that choice, even though it is made with love I still feel guilty. But one consolation is knowing that when the animals are ready to die, they tell us. Their spirits don't leave us; they stay with us through love, healing our lives and theirs.

Doreen's story, "My Boy Rusty," touched my heart. How many people stop to think about the mother dog? When you get a new puppy, you can send the puppy's mother a message of love; talk to her with your quiet mind and say, "We thank you; we love your puppy. We will be its father and its mother and take care of it for you. We'll send you messages so you know it's doing well."

When Rusty went to the nursing home he *was* giving therapy. The bonding hormones that are released when a woman nurses her baby are the same ones released when you pet a furry creature. It also helps people to bond with other people as they pet the dog and start talking to each other. If we all did more bonding with and caring for creatures, we'd have such a different world. Recognizing we're all divine, all the same color inside, we wouldn't be killing one another.

3

Love Is Blind

The wolf also shall dwell with the lamb, and the leopard shall lie down with the kid; and the calf and the young lion and the fatling together.

— Isaiah 11:6

In 2006, off the northwest coast of Ireland, an unusual friendship began. The carcass of a bottlenose dolphin washed up on the shores of Tory Island. Another dolphin, spotted close by, refused to leave the area. Whenever a school of dolphins passed, she'd go and swim with them for a while, but she always came back — alone. People assumed, since dolphins mate for life, that this pair had been partners. They named the solitary bottlenose Dougie.

It wasn't long before a local Labrador named Ben became enamored of the dolphin visitor. Every day he'd run down to the pier and wait. As soon as he saw Dougie, Ben would slip into the water and off they'd go, swimming and frolicking together. Ben's owner observed them playing together, often up to four hours a day. Sometimes Ben was so exhausted after a long session that the dolphin supported Ben's body with her nose while his tired legs pumped, and together they made their way back to the harbor.

No less remarkable was the devotion between a gray cat named Cheesy and a German shorthaired pointer named Oz. True buddies, they went everywhere together. When Oz's health seriously declined, his owner, Ali Le-Mar, called the vet to their home. After the doctor gave Oz a euthanizing injection, Ali showed the vet to the door. She went back inside to sit with her dog's body and found Cheesy the cat stretched across Oz's chest, where he remained, unmoving, for three hours.

When Cynthia's golden retriever Cherokee died, canine buddies Timber and Rosey sat and watched as their friend Jim dug the grave. The black barn cat who'd recently befriended Cherokee also joined them. All three animals remained stationed on or beside Cherokee's grave for the next two days. Their forlorn faces and slumped shoulders clearly expressed their sense of loss.

Sometimes we forget that the love between humans and their animals constitutes an interspecies relationship too. Our cat Miracle would follow me everywhere I went, even in the car. We'd go through the car wash, where she impressed the staff when she didn't act scared of the loud brushes and wasn't frightened by the sudsy water streaming down the windows. I could go into a store, leave her at the entrance, and she'd wait for me. She'd also walk on a leash, just like a dog.

One day a sign went up in our town: Dog Show. I put Miracle and our dog Furphy on leashes and took them to the show. When we arrived, the organizers said, "This is a dog show."

"She thinks she's a dog," I told them. "I'm not going to leave her at home and disappoint her." Miracle got so much attention, because all the dogs came over to sniff her; enormous dogs, like Newfoundlands, ran over, and she just sat there completely unafraid. People were saying, "Wow — look at that cat!" The next year a sign went up: Dog Show — *For Dogs Only.*

In the car, Miracle never slept but sat on the door next to my left arm, and I finally built a shelf there to make it more comfortable for her. She considered it her job to help me drive. On a twenty-hour, nonstop journey to Florida, with human and animal family members filling the car, Miracle sat on the dashboard and on her shelf and stayed awake the entire way to keep me alert and focused. Whenever she thought I was getting drowsy, she poked me. Of course this was back in the days before we realized the importance of seatbelts and safety cages or harnesses for animals. So don't do as I did; when you travel, remember to protect your animals just as would your children.

One time a plumber was at our house. He stood in front of me while explaining what he had to do and began waving his arms to demonstrate. Miracle suddenly jumped onto a table and flew at his waving arms. She thought he was threatening to hit me. At first the plumber and I were shocked and then amused. But I couldn't get over her courage. Here's this big guy, and she never thought he might toss her across the room; she only thought about protecting me.

Every day, heartwarming stories in the media confirm we are all interconnected. What affects one of us affects the others. These next stories of remarkable interspecies relationships show us the kind of love that transcends all barriers and eliminates boundaries.

Arlo's Lucky Dip

CYNTHIA J. HURN

≈≽≈

Arlo, at eleven, became my first senior golden retriever, filling my life with his gentle ways for eighteen precious months. In such a short time, he taught me an enormous amount about kindness, loving, and doing the right thing.

Every dawn we walked the trails alongside the American River. One day Arlo was off-leash and had gone several yards ahead of me when a beaver appeared on our path. Arlo and the beaver froze in their tracks and studied each other. Would either one of them attack the other? I held my breath, realizing I was too far away to intervene. Ever so slowly Arlo approached the beaver until they touched noses in a polite greeting. Arlo wagged his tail and the beaver turned, waddled down the bank, and slid into the river. Before I could get to Arlo, he loped down the bank and into the water! I called him back, but Arlo developed a sudden case of deafness as he swam with his new friend. For quite some time they frolicked like two boys on a hot summer's day. Perhaps twenty minutes passed before the beaver disappeared into his submerged den. Arlo paddled round and round, searching for his friend. Visibly disappointed, Arlo finally returned to his walk with me. Until the day he died, every time we passed that beaver's trail, Arlo would stop and gaze at the river, looking for his friend.

I fell in love with Arlo. I used to say that if he were

a man I'd marry him. He acted like his whole reason for living was my well-being. If Arlo didn't like the look of any man who approached us on our walk, he'd straddle the path and shield me with his great body, then stare at the man as if to say, she's mine, bud, so keep your distance. The stranger would get the message and give us a wide berth.

Arlo's passion for catching tennis balls — up to four at a time in his mouth — was surpassed only by his love for a soft blue teddy bear. At home, when my sweetheart gave me a hug, Arlo always wanted to join in. "Group hug!" he seemed to say with his glorious wagging tail. We'd wrap our arms around him and each other, making an Arlo sandwich. He'd beam at us with his four-ball-wide, golden-retriever grin: *this* was how life was meant to be!

When Arlo died, I had no place to put my grief. I just didn't know what to do with it. But even in death Arlo taught me about love, transforming my grief into something beautiful. Two days after he died, I returned Arlo's unused medications to the rescue center and came home with Shadow, another senior golden, whose need for a loving family was the same shape and size as the void Arlo had left behind.

While I was delighted to have Shadow in my life, I didn't want to forget a single moment with Arlo. I took a sheet of paper and wrote down words and short phrases that described my experience of him. I cut them out, folded the strips of paper, and placed them in a bowl beside the cedar box that contained Arlo's ashes. Whenever a previously forgotten scene of Arlo popped into my mind, I'd add a few more words to the bowl.

Anytime I felt the pang of loss, I'd stir up the pieces of paper and pick one out. As I unfolded the paper slip I'd find a little bit of Arlo in those words. Instead of increasing my grief, the lucky-dip memories increased my gratitude for having had such a good spirit in my life. Feeling comforted, I'd replace the folded paper with a quiet "Thank you, Arlo."

Two years later our neighbor's dog, Bingo, had to be put down. Arlo had adored Bingo, and now, so did Shadow. I wanted to offer my neighbor some comfort or support, but I was at a loss for words. I went to Arlo's pot, asked for his guidance, and pulled out a piece of paper. Arlo made it crystal clear what I needed to do.

Shadow and I went over to my neighbor's house and gave her the piece of paper, telling her it was from Arlo's pot. She unfolded it, read the message, and with tears in her eyes, opened her arms to me and Shadow. On the paper were two words: *Group hug.*

Interconnection of Nature

Geoff Johnson

≈≈

I was just a rugby-playing cow vet living on the edge of Exmoor, in South West England, when I first heard about homeopathy. I had suffered all my life from the sort of hay fever that makes your eyes so itchy you just want to claw them out, and I had taken antihistamines for years, until one June when I went camping and forgot to bring them. I was in a horrible state, but it may have been one of the luckiest things that ever happened to me, because five tents away was a woman who was a homeopath.

I was encouraged to go and see her. For twenty minutes she asked me totally irrelevant questions that, as far as I could see, had nothing to do with hay fever. At the end of her questioning, she gave me one pill.

"How many do I take per day and for how many days?" I asked.

"You just take the one pill," she said.

"But surely, I must have more," I insisted.

"Just take the one," she responded calmly. "You might be an expert veterinarian, but I'm an expert homeopath."

To my astonishment, half an hour after taking the remedy, my hay fever was 90 percent better. From that day in 1995, I have not taken another antihistamine.

For me, this was impossible, going against everything I learned in six years' veterinary training at Cambridge. I couldn't understand *how* this had happened, but it *had* happened, so I had to explore homeopathy and find out how it worked. My education began all over again.

Now I run a homeopathy-only practice and give nutritional advice. I absolutely love it. It's taught me so many things. I'm not reading only veterinary manuals; I'm reading about philosophy, quantum physics, and the nature of plants and their environment. That's where all the remedies come from. In order to choose the best remedy, you need to understand its origin, habitat, traits, and function in the natural world.

This study reconnected me to my earliest love. The reason I became a vet was because of my love for nature and animals. To be able to treat an unhappy dog, a depressed horse, or an aggressive cow suffering an unpleasant physical ailment, and to see that animal, over a period of days to weeks, get miraculously better, especially when all other treatments failed — there's no greater feeling and nothing I'd rather do.

My love for animals, and the study of this new form of medicine, brought me to an even deeper understanding about our interconnectedness. One day I was called to an organic dairy farm. The white-blood-cell count in the milk was reaching illegal levels. A high cell count is an indication of chronic mastitis in the herd; it must stay below four hundred thousand cells per millimeter or the milk cannot be sold.

Twelve months previously the cell count was two hundred thousand — perfectly acceptable. It then began to rise, and no homeopathic or conventional treatment would control it. Why? Disease is *always* there for a reason.

I individually examined three cows whose cell counts were too high and treated them with three homeopathic remedies for this condition. Suspecting there was more going on here, I sat down with the farmer and went through the farmer's recent history, knowing that the health of a herd is intimately related to the health of the farmer.

The farmer had previously developed numbness and coldness in his feet, which proved to be arteriosclerosis of his femoral arteries; he'd undergone an operation and taken three months off work. His wife, an ambitious woman and famous textile designer, had organized the building of an organic restaurant at the farm, hoping to attract people to see the textiles and bring more income to the family. This had upset the farmer considerably.

"The builders just come without asking and move things around that I don't want moved. I feel my home is invaded. It's hard for my wife too; they bully her, and I can't do anything about it."

"What is this experience like for you?" I asked.

"I feel powerless, like a small boy in shorts at school. I've let my wife down; I should be in charge of everything, but the builders just don't listen."

"What makes you feel better?" was my next question.

"Being with my cows — I go and stand with them in the field — and getting into my normal routine with my cows."

The farmer's answers identified key elements in the overall picture. The farmer felt that his lack of control over the builders was his fault, and he lacked power to deal with the situation, suggesting that a problem or lack lay within him. There were also issues related to home and routine, and his feelings were ameliorated when he spent time with his cows. His feeling like a small boy, and his condition of arteriosclerosis, were also markers that led to the appropriate homeopathic treatment for him.

I elected to give *his* remedy to every animal on the farm daily for three days and then once weekly. An aqueous solution was put into the drinking troughs and sprayed on the cows in the milking parlor. The farmer would receive his treatment while being drenched by the spray.

The worried farmer phoned me three days later; the cell count had gone from 400,000 to 670,000. I hoped this was an aggravation, a not uncommon sign that the right remedy had been administered but at too high a dose. I told him to stop dosing and wait. The cell count then started to fall, eventually reaching a healthy 180,000 over three months, where it has remained for the past year.

This and similar cases demonstrate that farm animals can be affected by events in the farmer's life. We are all beings of energy, and nothing exists in isolation. When a group is linked by the elements of nature, care, and love, it is totally valid to regard that group as a single being, whether they are of the same species or not. That the cows healed by taking the farmer's remedy was no miracle, unless you recognize that life is a miracle in itself.

An Interspecies Affair

Mookie, my red-eared slider turtle, had suddenly stopped eating. Not only that, but she just didn't look interested in her surroundings. We called our vet, who explained that Mookie had entered her adolescent years and she wanted to hunt, just as she would in the wild. Nature had designed her to enjoy certain activities, and without these, life was no fun anymore.

"Provide her with feeder fish," he advised, and so we drove to the pet supply store. As we stood in front of tanks filled with shining goldfish, guppies, and minnows, Mom was visibly experiencing some conflict.

"I don't want *Animal Kingdom* happening in our living room," she said, "but we love Mookie…and we do want her to be well…and it is up to us to make sure she's got everything she needs…"

Finding the resolve to do a heinous deed for the sake of our beloved turtle, Mom asked a store employee to get *one* fish out of the tank.

"You should get a dozen," he said, visibly annoyed.

"We only want one in case something goes wrong," I said. The sales clerk rolled his eyes and scooped one thirteen-cent feeder fish out with a net.

As we carried the fish home in a little plastic bag, we couldn't make eye contact with him, knowing we were bringing him to his watery grave. Our tradition has always been to name all members of our family, regardless of which species they belong to. But this little fish's fate was already sealed; and somehow, giving him a name before throwing him into the lion's den, so to speak, was something we just couldn't do. So we put him in the tank and called him "Mr. Fishy," a respectful yet impersonal solution.

About thirty seconds after Mr. Fishy entered the tank, Mookie realized she was not alone. Not sure of this new creature at first, she watched him for a moment, then darted toward him as if planning to gulp him down in one bite. It seemed the dreaded event of nature was going to occur in our living room, like it or not. We braced ourselves for that awful moment when Mr. Fishy would disappear.

Mookie swam straight up to Mr. Fishy and stopped, turtle snout to fish nose. At five inches long, Mookie seemed enormous compared to the one-inch goldfish. We held our breath as an odd expression filled her eyes. It certainly wasn't the stare of a hunter. She blinked. They studied each other for a moment, then, much to our surprise, they simply turned and swam around the tank, like Mutt and Jeff in a pond.

Never having seen a turtle hunt, we weren't sure how long Mr. Fishy would be allowed to live. Each morning we switched on the aquarium light, prepared to find Mookie alone in the tank, but that day never came. Day after day, Mr. Fishy swam right alongside Mookie.

Mookie's appetite returned. She started eating about two days after her tank mate moved in. Mr. Fishy would swim up to the surface, helping himself to turtle pellets while Mookie grazed in her typical contented way at the other end of the tank. As time went on, they became so comfortable with each other that Mr. Fishy would eat right alongside Mookie, without showing any signs of fear. When Mookie climbed up on her floating dock to bask in the sunlight, Mr. Fishy would swim underneath it and suck the dead scales off her feet, which were dangling in the water. When the spa treatment was over, she'd slide back into the tank; Mr. Fishy would make way for her, then catch up to her and swim alongside.

They became the best of friends. Even when Mookie ate shrimp, tearing at it with her sharp claws, Mr. Fishy would stick his head right into her mouth, helping himself to torn bits of crustacean delight, seemingly confident that she wouldn't retaliate. And she never did.

Whenever soul mates come together and care for one another, their bond brings joy into the lives of the people who witness this love in action. We never dreamed the "animal kingdom" in our living room would become such a magical event — a turtle and a fish making their tank and our home a place of remarkable love.

Color-Blind

DORIE WALDEN

It was a warm sunny day, and I took a break from my chores to relax in the backyard. I put my chair where I could take advantage of a gentle breeze blowing from the south. As I sat mentally listing the work I still had to do, a flash of movement caused me to look up. A pair of birds flew past and landed in a tree at the back of the yard. With so many trees and flowers on the property, we get lots of birds, so I don't know why this particular pair caught and held my attention. They weren't even near enough for me to see them clearly, but I found myself sitting very still, hoping they'd fly closer, close enough for me to observe them.

Within a few minutes, the pair flew down to a spot adjacent to me on the lawn. They were identical except that one bird was black and the other pure white. They began to forage for food and chattered constantly as they scratched, jabbed, and thrust their beaks into the lawn. I noticed that the black bird stayed close to the white one, and he seemed to be helping the white bird locate his meal. The black bird would take a bite and then gently nudge the other bird's beak toward the food.

Every time they flew to a new spot, they remained close together and continued chirping as they traveled, seeming to function as a unit. They worked harmoni-ously as the white bird seemed to trust and follow the black bird's prompts. When they finished their meal, the birds flew away, still staying very near to each other. Sadly, I never saw them again.

My guess is that the white bird was an albino and, probably blind, had become dependent on its partner. The black bird demonstrated such devotion to the albino, pushing food his way and maintaining a constant bridge of sound. It must have been hard work for the black bird, thinking not only of his own needs but also of those of his companion.

In those few minutes I witnessed one of nature's lessons in the true meaning of compassion, patience, and love. Such a simple demonstration by two birds touched my heart and made me realize we are all capable of creating miracles when we go out of our way to meet the needs of another.

Bear Mountain

Sonia S. Wolshin

⁖

Whenever *she* came to stay at our cabin on Bear Mountain, I got lots of hugs, love, and attention. He didn't fuss over me that much. Don't get me wrong; he'd give me the odd scratch behind my ears or on my back, just above my tail, and let me curl up beside him when he stared at the noise box. He'd let me out to roam, sometimes for five hours or more, until I scratched on the door. I'd explore the mountain, play catch with a camper at the lake, or scare off the coyote packs that tease campers' dogs. There were bears around too; as long as I respected them, we'd nod at each other and move on.

She'd come and go like a butterfly. She'd get up at dawn to walk me and then go snowboarding alone; he'd wake hours later and drive me in his truck down to the place where he eats breakfast. I had to wait on the porch, but I always got a pat on the head from the locals. When he drove us home he'd turn on the noise box and leave it blaring all day. I'd sit outside waiting for her to come back and hike with me again. She only ever stayed for two to three months at a time; and each time she left, I'd pine for days, hoping that the next time she came she'd just stay.

One day when she wasn't staying with us, he forgot to tie me up before he went down the mountain. He often left me chained outside for two days, with food and water nearby. It was a challenge to fight off animal intruders while tied to a stake. This time I followed him. I ran as fast as I could down the mountain, but I couldn't keep up with his truck. I heard the locals yelling, "Stop!" But I kept running, hoping I'd catch him. Finally I couldn't run anymore; then someone else saw me, and I ended up in a cold, scary place with a bunch of other sad animals.

I hoped he would come and get me, but he didn't. Every night that he didn't show up, I grew more and more scared. When he finally came, I showed him how glad I was to see him, but he wasn't acting happy to see me. I curled up next to him on the seat anyway. I was tired and not feeling so great. This was going to be a long ride home.

A while later he stopped the truck. I didn't smell the mountain. I smelled ocean. That's when I caught the scent of her! I nearly turned inside out as I ran straight into her arms. It seemed that I was to stay with her for good. Now he was just my bud, and she was my LOVE.

She gave me my new name, Lady Girl, and I thought of her as "She Who Loves." She took me everywhere and introduced me to people who gave me treats — Joey at the post office, Zelda at the bank, and Sarah and Mary at the store. I never dreamed life could be this good. She never left me to fend for myself, and she always showed me that I was loved. She took me up to Big Bear to visit with my old bud on occasion, but I'd stick by her side. We'd walk down to the lake in the mornings and hike the trail above at dusk. Animals recognized her as a native medicine woman, a healer who loves all animals, and they trusted her. Even bears stopped to visit with her on our hikes.

One day she was singing on our way back from a long hike. I picked up the scent of bear, but this time I knew we were in danger; this was the scent of bear *cubs*. I stopped in my tracks hoping she'd stop too, but she kept walking and calling, "Chase the stick, Lady Girl. Go get it!" I ignored her calls, hoping she'd realize something was wrong, but she didn't get it. In desperation, I ran over and sat on her toes. She kept moving and pulled me by the collar. I even skidded on my butt, trying to stop her. *Finally* she stopped.

"What's wrong, girl?" That's when she saw the two bear cubs up a tree, right next to the creek we needed to cross to get home.

Yes! Yes! I wagged as she kneeled down and put her arm around me. But when she didn't stop talking, saying, "Look! They're so beautiful...," my heart sank. We were too close to them for comfort. I stared at her with the most intense look I could, for now I was picking up the scent of the momma bear. She Who Loves couldn't smell who was coming. She just kept watching those cubs and cooing, making me more frightened for her than ever.

At last she went silent. I had my back to the cubs, and I could tell by her face she'd spotted the momma bear. Now I could hear the bear running down the mountain, barreling toward her cubs — and us. She Who Loves froze, but her heart was racing and I could smell her fear. "Don't run," I was thinking to her. I stared into her eyes and used my gaze to calm her heartbeat down.

We did not move a muscle for the fifteen minutes it took that momma bear to get her cubs down out of the tree. Luckily for us, the bear took no offense if she caught our scent. She and the cubs went on their way — in the other direction.

I later listened to She Who Loves telling people how Lady Girl saved her life, but the truth is, she, who loves like no other, saved my life — over and over again.

Bernie's Comments

In "Arlo's Lucky Dip," we see animals enjoying their commonality, not fighting over their differences. If we only learned that lesson from them, there'd be no reason or room for war.

In the same way that Arlo and the beaver communicated, the dog's spirit communicated with Cynthia, for consciousness is never-ending. What died was the body. Consciousness can be relayed through words, symbols, images, a song, or an object. Cynthia's dad once told her that after his death, she should look for a bald eagle; that would be him. A few months after she moved to California he died, but there were no eagles living in her area. She worried about how she would know her dad was okay. Then, out of the blue, somebody sent her a present, and it was an eagle kite with a red heart on its breast. That gift was her dad saying, "I'm here, and I love you. My spirit's not dead." Arlo was saying the same thing.

In Geoff Johnson's story, "Interconnection of Nature," it's nice to see someone who was trained scientifically, keeping an open mind, seeking further education, and doing what he does now.

When I developed Lyme disease and other problems, homeopathy was recommended to me, and I tried it. I don't think the positive result I experienced was a placebo effect; I approached homeopathy with a skeptical, but open, mind — more as an experiment. And I saw the benefits. Even if I can't explain why it works, I'm still open to using it.

Treating the farmer and the animals as one patient makes sense. We are all one. When the farmer is treated, the cows sense that, and they get better sooner. It's similar to when I raise my voice and Bobbie says, "Honey, you're upsetting the animals." When I'm upset about something, it affects them. If I calm down, then they don't worry, and they feel better too.

Charlie Siegel is our grandson. When you read about the animals in his story, "An Interspecies Affair," you see mixed species — a turtle and a fish. Neither of them is killing the other, and both of them are taking care of each other. Hunting is part of their instinct to survive, and it must be enjoyable to some extent. But love is much more important to them, as shown by the turtle. Mookie had something to eat; she didn't need to hunt, but what she did need was to give and receive love. We were meant to get along together and share this world with each other, to meet the others' needs and live in peace. Even turtles and fish become our teachers and healers. This story is a wonderful lesson for life: the biggest lesson of all is that *we are all family*.

Dorie Walden's "Color-Blind" reminds me of another story, in which a person went to heaven and saw several angels with only one wing. He asked his guide, "How does a one-winged angel fly?" The guide said, "Watch." Two angels, each with only one wing, linked arms and flew off together. I have heard numerous accounts of blind and deaf animals being guided through life by another animal of a different species.

Cynthia Hurn once witnessed a "rook's parliament." A group of black crows formed a circle around a pure white crow (the offender) and were screaming accusations at the albino bird. After a raucous verbal onslaught, the birds went silent; the offender was condemned. The black crows proceeded, one by one, to attack the albino and would have pecked him to death had his human observer not chased the executioners away.

The crows' collective behavior reflects nature's way of eliminating weak genes, making Dorie's story even more remarkable, for a normally colored bird would seem to have little reason to help the albino bird.

These two birds are good role models for us. We need to stop, help the needy, and converse with them. To someone who is blind, another person's voice can be a lifeline. To someone living on the street, ignored by people who pass by, attention given by a stranger is assurance that they are still valuable. I always feel good when I stop and talk with the homeless. So take time to give someone your attention. Be a one-winged angel.

In "Bear Mountain," the dog adores the woman who spends time taking her for long walks. Two of the most valuable gifts we can give to each other, whether human or animal, are time and affection. I have always loved the peace I gain when walking with my dogs and cat. And they love going on excursions with their tribe. Animals know when we are in danger, and this dog responded to the situation appropriately, neither chasing after the bear nor barking and alerting her to their position. Lady Girl's greatest desire was to protect and be with the person she loved. She focused on her love rather than on the problem, and the dog's desire came true.

4

Reverence for Life

A work of art crossed my path
A red squirrel
A better artist than Picasso created him
My heart was changed by this creature
He has something I will never achieve
Perfection in form, movement, life
I look for him everywhere in the hope we will meet
I want to feed him and sustain his beauty
To offer him a treat
The world needs its red squirrels
They are complete

— Bernie Siegel

When I was a boy, I listened to the stories of my grandfather, who, in his earlier years, had taught Judaism in Russia. He was walking to his class when Cossacks, riding their horses through town, saw him, rode over, and tried to split his head open with a saber. My grandfather got away. I used to think the story was too extreme to be true, until I went to medical school. At Bellevue Hospital in New York, I came upon a patient who had a deep V in the center of his head. I asked him what happened.

"When I was a kid in Russia the Cossacks tried to kill me," he said. "I was in the street, and they split my head open with a sword."

This indentation went down a couple of inches into his head. The skin had healed over it, obviously, but I don't know how a kid could survive that kind of wound. After hearing his story and seeing the brutal results, I realized what my grandfather had gone through.

Years later, I remembered that patient and my reaction — how horrible that somebody would do that — when I learned *I had done it* in a previous life. My lord had commanded me to kill the daughter of his enemy. I asked, "If I don't kill this girl, what will you do?" His reply was: "I'll kill you." So I killed her out of fear for my own life. Her dog, who tried to protect her, also became a victim of my sword. During my visualization of that past-life scene, I approached the young woman with my sword, and she looked into my eyes with such a look. I was shocked to recognize her as the woman I am married to today. From the moment Bobbie and I met, her eyes have always had an amazing effect on me. I have never been able to stay angry with her when she looks at me. I just feel love.

It was little to do with faith, but more with this experience of my past life, which caused my current life to become a spiritual journey, shaving the head, and why I

explored a whole host of things that I had no prior understanding of. I began to read the works of, and talk to, enlightened people. The more I learned, the more reverence
for life I gained, and I found a lord I could have faith in.

In the days when I went to medical school, we didn't
have computerized virtual anatomy labs, and it affected
me deeply to cut open live animals and study their insides. One day I read a poem that told the story of a soldier who returned from the war to go to medical school.
When he was overseas, a dog named Rags had served
with his unit and saved many lives. The soldier wanted
to bring the dog home, but couldn't find him when he
was being discharged. He figured they must have sent the
animal home already.

In the poem the young man gets to medical school,
goes into the laboratory for a lecture, and there's a dog
lying on the table; he's been cut open, and the medical
students are all walking by for the anatomy lesson. The
man realizes it is Rags displayed on that table. He goes
over to him; Rags sees him, whines, licks his hand, and
dies. Rags forgave the hands that killed him. The poet
says, "And if there's no Heaven for love like that...if I
have any choice...I'll take my chance in hell." That poem
brought me to tears. If animals can love us like that, how
can we not respond with a reverence for all life?

The following stories deal with irreverence, its ugly
head, and some of the repercussions. They also reveal
that beautiful things happen when people with reverence
for life change the world of one animal or that of a whole
species.

Nameless

Terri Crisp

꩜

During a major flood in Georgia, I managed a disaster rescue team that gave temporary safe shelter to animals whose owners were forced to evacuate. At one house a man claimed to have two dogs. When we offered to take them to the shelter, he shrugged his shoulders.

"Makes no difference to me."

I convinced him to get the dogs. He crawled under the elevated porch of his dilapidated house, hauled out a black-and-white dog, dragged it to my truck, and shoved him in a crate. He never spoke a word to the dog as he walked away.

"Does he have a name?" asked Amy, one of the rescue team.

"Nope," he replied.

Unable to locate the other dog, we returned to the shelter. When Amy opened the crate's door, the dog sat, head lowered. Amy tried coaxing him out, but he wouldn't budge. Finally, she slipped a leash around the dog's neck, and slowly raised the back end of the crate. The animal slid out, landed on the grass, and just lay there.

"I'm guessing he's been abused," Amy said, shaking her head sadly. "The first thing I'm doing for you," she told the dog, "is give you a name. From now on, you're Albert."

For the next two days the sixty-pound Albert refused

to move. When Amy fed the other dogs, she'd pick up Albert and move him along, keeping him with her. In spite of all the barking and commotion around him, Albert didn't react. He just sat, staring at the ground. We ended up borrowing a golf cart. When Amy made her feeding rounds, Albert sat in the front seat of the cart, his eyes fixed on the floorboard.

At night Albert lay next to Amy's cot. During meals he sat beside her, refusing any of the human food offered to him. In the afternoons, Amy found a shady spot and stretched out on the ground next to Albert. I watched her whispering into Albert's ear and could only imagine what she was saying to the lifeless dog.

Albert had been with us for four days when we had a late-night birthday party for one of the volunteers. There were outbursts of laughter, much storytelling, and lots of cake being consumed. Seated in the middle of the festivities was Amy and, close beside her, the unresponsive Albert.

"Look!" a volunteer shouted above the clamor. He pointed at Albert. The whole group went silent. For the first time since he'd arrived, the tip of Albert's tail was quivering. We stared in amazement as Albert's entire tail slowly began to wag. Finally he stood up, his rear end switching back and forth as if someone had suddenly pushed Albert's on-button.

The once nameless dog never stopped wagging from that day forward. And he always remained a step behind Amy. Now when she made her feeding rounds, Albert trotted along, barking at the other dogs as if to say, "I'm happy." When Amy walked to the nearby fire station to take a shower, Albert went too. When Amy got in the shower, Albert hopped right in, refusing to let her out of his sight.

Despite his new buoyancy, Albert's display of energy was still far too low. A visit to the vet confirmed that Albert had heartworms. The good news was that Albert's young age meant the treatment had more likelihood of success.

I called Albert's owner to explain that his dog had heartworms and that the treatment cost three hundred dollars. I expected he'd say, "Keep the dog. I don't have that kind of money." But I was wrong. The man wanted Albert back.

"You understand if the dog isn't treated he'll die," I said, still hoping I could convince him to release the dog to me.

"Yep. That's what happens to all my dogs. When one goes, I get another one," he replied with no remorse. That's when the hammer fell.

"My house never did flood. I'll be by shortly to get my dog." And he hung up.

Amy and Albert were playing tug-of-war with a towel. I watched them as tears streamed down my cheeks. How was I going to tell Amy we had to give Albert back?

An hour later a car pulled up. The man got out carrying a heavy, rusted chain. I had already explained to Amy that Albert's owner was coming to get him. Fighting tears, Amy had taken Albert for a final walk.

"Where's my dog?" the man demanded.

"He's being walked," I replied. I could see Amy over his shoulder as she crouched next to Albert, her arms wrapped around his neck. This time I knew what she was whispering in his ear. She was saying good-bye.

"Well, go an' get him. I don' got all day!" Turning to look for his dog, the man said, "There he is," and strode off toward Amy.

"Wait!" I blurted out. "Can I buy your dog?" I held my breath as I waited for his answer.

"Hell, yeah!"

The man left with only his rusted chain and $50 in his pocket.

Albert would never live under a porch again. The heartworm treatment was successful, and he became a valuable member of Amy's family. After a lifetime filled with fun, love, and kindness, the dog that had once been so unvalued, died. Engraved on his memorial was his name, Happy Albert.

Tokitae

SANDRA POLLARD

~≈~

They call me Lolita now, but my real name is Tokitae. In Coast Salish language it means "nice day, pretty colors." The Salish Sea is home to the southern resident orcas in summer, our season for hunting Chinook salmon. It was in the cool, temperate waters of the Pacific Northwest, from southern British Columbia to the northernmost tip of Washington State, where I roamed before I was stolen, made captive, and imprisoned.

My family lived in harmony, staying together for life, sharing food, and caring for one another. But men in boats chased us and threw explosives into the water to frighten and disorient us. They herded us into coves from which we could not escape, trapped us in nets, and separated us from our mothers before transporting us thousands of miles away.

In August 1970, my family of more than a hundred whales was driven into Penn Cove on Whidbey Island. Terrified and confused by the violence inflicted upon us, four of my playmates died. When the men in black strapped me to a skiff and dragged me away, I screamed and cried. My mother cried too and tried to follow, but she was helpless to save me. None of the humans listened to our cries.

There were strange noises and sensations I'd never experienced. I was lifted from the water by an iron monster that jerked and shook me. I was torn from the source of all life I'd ever known — the ocean — dropped onto a flatbed truck, and driven to an aquarium in Seattle. A veterinarian checked my vital signs, saying I would be perfect for the Miami Sea Aquarium.

I could no longer hear my mother's calls, and I wondered when I would return to my family. Soon my heart filled with terror again as I was pushed into the cargo hold of an airplane, thrust skyward, away from home and all I had ever known.

That happened forty-four years ago. It's been a long time since I had a "nice day, pretty colors," a good day of hunting and enjoying my ocean home. Now I perform tricks to loud music for humans who scream and shout. Twice a day somebody rides on my back and stands on my nose to "rocket hop." Clapping, the watchers call, "Lolita, Lolita!" They don't know that's my stage name, that my real name was changed to avoid awkward questions about my origins. They don't know where I came from; they don't even ask. When the show is over, my trainer feeds me dead fish. It keeps my body alive, but the hunger that tears at my heart and soul is never appeased.

The shows take up one hour of my day. For the rest of the time I am alone. My pod mate, Hugo, died in 1980. I haven't seen any other members of my family since I was taken.

It is hot in Miami. There's no shelter from the sun, which blazes down on my tiny tank. The deep ocean used to protect my skin, but now I am covered in zinc oxide to prevent sunburn. I spend hours and hours just lying on the surface of the pool. There's nothing else to do, nowhere else to go.

I haven't forgotten my family. One day this cursed existence *will* come to an end. Somebody came here and played to me a recording of unique orca calls. I recognized the language of L-pod, my own family unit, and of the other two pods, named J and K. Immediately memories came flooding back…of foraging among kelp beds, exploring around rocks, playing and roaming up to a hundred miles a day, and swimming in my mother's slipstream. The conversations and songs of the other whales enveloped me in the knowledge of who I am. I was only four or five years old when they kidnapped me, but I remember. I remember.

Only eighty members of my family, the southern resident community, remain. We are classed as an endangered species, culturally and genetically distinct from other orcas. I was excluded from the listing, for I am still in this prison aquarium.

Men in boats and airplanes abducted around forty members of my family and killed thirteen others in Washington State waters during the brutal capture era between 1965 and 1976. My cousin Corky, captured in Canadian waters, and I are the sole survivors of that terrible era. The others, who were torn from our fragile community, all died in captivity by 1987.

They are not forgotten. Every year a commemoration is held in Penn Cove to remember those of us stolen from our homeland waters. And this year Washington State launched a new ferry, named Tokitae to honor my memory. I have heard that many kindhearted, determined people, including a team of dedicated lawyers, are fighting for my freedom. If the courts recognize my right to a free existence and to not be forced to perform stupid tricks in return for dead fish, I will no longer be put on public display. The show will finally be over.

These people say that *when* I regain my freedom, the plans that are already in place to move me to a sea pen, close to where my family passes by, will be set in motion. I will hear their calls again after so many years of longing, and they will finally hear mine.

My mother must be in her eighties now, so I hope it won't be long. When I am strong enough to swim with her, they will release me from the sea pen. My mother's breath will merge with mine as we breach the waves and hunt in the Salish Sea. Spy hops, tail lobs, cartwheels, and pectoral fin waves — mother and child will join in the ancient dance of Orca, together at last, and *free*.

The Stowaway

ANONYMOUS

≈≈

It all started as it would end — with a cardboard box. My husband and I had just returned from our honeymoon when rumors of trouble on the sleeper train from Newton Abbot, Devon, to Sterling, Scotland, began to come in. My husband, a brand-new and very green area manager for British Rail, went to investigate reports of cat noises emanating from the train floor. Each time the train returned from Scotland, another round of passengers complained, so the inspector from the Royal Society for the Prevention of Cruelty to Animals, with the help of station staff, would search the train. Cat traps were set and undercarriages flushed with hoses, but nothing ever appeared.

The determined inspector took four round-trips to Scotland before locating the tiny kitten deep inside the train's undercarriage. After giving birth while the train was parked on a siding, the kitten's mother probably jumped off when the train moved, leaving her orphan, frozen with fear, to ride the rails. The wrong side of the tracks is a tough beginning for any ruffian, but the tracks themselves are even worse.

The inspector reached in to grab the kitten and quickly withdrew a severely shredded hand. After a remarkable show of combative determination, the kitten fell into the inspection pit below and was captured. A

74

pulsating cardboard box was then deposited on my husband's desk. The inspector assured him that this wild kitten would never be domesticated, and he offered to destroy the animal. But my husband decided to bring the kitten home, instead. He deserved a chance at life, and the poor thing hadn't had much of a chance so far.

We gingerly opened the box to a volley of curses. Guarding the corner was a bristling mass of furious black with glaring yellow eyes. He was so small we wondered whether he'd even been weaned. We offered him milk, but he refused it. We tried a little meat, and he accepted this, making sounds of famished desperation. He was so weak he could not stand, and we feared he wouldn't survive the night, but there was little more we could do.

The next morning the kitten was alive, but his temper had not improved. All the overtures we made were met with furious hissing; he even managed to bite through industrial leather gloves that we'd borrowed from the rail workers. Pathetically thin, the poor kitten was still unable to stand. I telephoned my mother, an expert on reviving waifs and strays. She advised that we must get the thick layer of engine oil out of his coat before he tried to wash himself, or he wouldn't survive.

I cautiously opened the box and was ordered in a belligerent treble to go away. Persevering, I managed to grab the oily creature and lower him into a basin of warm water. Suddenly the curses stopped. He became quite still.

My heart sank. Was this one shock too many for his beleaguered little body? Several seconds passed before I realized he was purring. For some wonderful reason he decided to submit to whatever treatment was necessary and trust me. When my husband returned from work the much cleaner and attractively marked black-and-white kitten swore halfheartedly at him, then spent the evening nestled into his neck.

It was a week before the kitten could stand unaided, and several years before he'd stay in the room, or even the house, with anyone other than us. Our friends and family refused to believe he existed, because he vanished the minute he heard strange footsteps. He did make an exception for my mother, becoming quite friendly toward her.

At first we named him Sabbry (an acronym for "Scotland and back by railway"), but he came to be called Kitten Bear and, when he reached maturity, KB. He grew into a fine muscular animal and devoted family cat. KB traveled regularly with us by train, but in rather more comfort than on his original journey.

At night, particularly in his later years, he slept between us with his head on the pillow, his back braced against one human and his legs against the other, maintaining ownership of his space. KB's greatest display of affection was to bite your nose. Many times in the night we would wake to Kitten Bear, overcome with emotion, chewing hard.

With implicit faith that we could make him better, he always brought his injuries to us, bearing all treatment with dignity and stoicism. He braved broken legs and battle wounds with equanimity, and he defended his patch with determination, relying heavily on his rich vocabulary. Whether he swore in Devonian or Scots we shall never know.

After seventeen years, KB's kidneys failed. It was a hot July evening when we took him to the vet for the last time. His heart was so strong it required a double dose. We brought him home in a cardboard box, wrapped in one of my husband's old sweaters. Tearfully we dug a hole for him in the garden and discovered a perfectly square piece of white marble. In return for a bottle of Jack Daniels, a monumental mason inscribed it: KB 1972–1989.

About thirteen years later, we moved to a derelict house in the country. It was a huge, daunting project. The house was close to collapse, extremely cold, and damp. One day I was feeling miserable, cold, and exhausted. I had a nasty kidney infection and lay on my bed feeling sorry for myself. Suddenly I was aware of a weight on the bed beside me. Then I heard a gentle, yet unmistakable purr. Since there were no animals on the farm yet, I realized it was KB's spirit. This time he had come to comfort me.

Captiva the Dolphin

JANET ELIZABETH COLLI

≈

I was dying of cancer when I had the dream. A poster on the bulletin board at the swimming pool announced I would be facilitating encounters between dolphins and cancer patients. Awakening with the certainty that I was meant to live gave me the courage to fight. I not only lived, I flourished.

Two years after the dream, I traveled from Seattle to the Florida Keys simply to explore the meaning of it. After all, I owed my life to dolphins, and I was determined to find out why. As I stood on the dock at the Dolphin Research Center, the tour guide introduced us to the residents. I could easily tell Captiva apart from the other dolphins. Never mind her bulging right eye; the celebrated dolphin smile that graces every other dolphin's lips was grotesquely transformed on Captiva's. Her lower jaw hung permanently askew. Her lips did not meet, and her front teeth were covered with green algae. To the casual observer, Captiva had a face only a mother could love. So why was it love at first sight for me?

My introduction to this member of a species known for its symmetry, grace, and beauty affected me in a different way, with compassion. This dolphin touched my heart. Having been diagnosed with cancer at thirty, I was no casual observer. I knew what it was to be singled out for suffering. Not surprisingly, the guide remarked, when cancer survivors visited the center, Captiva was always their favorite dolphin.

Named for the island where she was caught, Captiva had been fated to become a show dolphin at an aquarium. But her right eye developed an infection that left her with a blind, bulging eye. With her career nipped in the bud, she'd been transported to the Dolphin Research Center. Captiva was just getting used to her new home when she appeared one morning with a severely broken jaw. Perhaps she slammed into a dock when pursued by Natua, the dominant male. Shy Captiva had been noticeably put off by his advances. Regardless of the accident's cause, Captiva's ability to trust would be shattered anew when undergoing the medical treatment for saving her life.

The tour guide droned on, but my attention was riveted on the broken-jawed dolphin as I felt a jolt of recognition. She was a survivor, just like me. Moreover, Captiva had been the first dolphin in the world to endure that invasive medical procedure. This dolphin, sashaying through the waters right before my eyes, fulfilled every cancer patient's dream: she had made medical history and survived against all odds.

Most of the dolphins savored an occasional touch. But this was no petting pool; the natural lagoon afforded plenty of swim space. Moreover, a high degree of trust and familiarity was necessary before the dolphins permitted anyone to touch them. But Captiva simply would not swim close enough to the dock to be touched.

My first day on the dock was largely spent trying to

entice her to come closer. No amount of coaxing would convince her. Instead, my boundless enthusiasm evolved into a healthy respect for her boundaries. Our interaction developed into an elaborate game of peek-a-boo. Captiva would torpedo through the water only to stop a couple of feet short of the dock.

"There she is!" I'd cry. Captiva would do a double take then dive under the dock only to surface on the other side. When I'd leave the dock and hide behind a post, she'd watch curiously, maintaining eye contact. Captiva's consciousness wasn't just on the water. It was on the dock and on the paths, seeking mine.

I sensed that her evolved consciousness had developed in part because of her operation. After all, the scars from being wounded in the war against cancer had forced me to work extra hard to make a connection with others too. Paradoxically, my greatest growth resulted from contact with the realm of doctors, chemotherapy, and radiation. I resolved to find out more about the operation that had rendered Captiva virtually untouchable yet had left her with a mind capable of intimate contact.

The operation had been recorded on video. I watched the entire two-hour ordeal. No scene could depict helpless terror more than a dolphin out of water, struggling on an operating table, surrounded by humans wielding sharp instruments. General anesthesia was out of the question. Dolphins are conscious breathers; if they fall completely asleep, they die. The surgeon dared only to use mild painkillers.

The operation involved resetting broken bones in her

lower jaw and fitting a brace to hold them in place until they healed. Dolphins' jaws enable echolocation when sound waves strike the jawbone and travel to the inner eardrum. Seven stainless steel screws for the brace were *drilled* through this exquisitely sensitive nerve tissue. Captiva's mouth gushed blood like a fountain.

Horrified, I could hardly stand to watch. I too had been on that operating table. I faced my own death once more by identifying with Captiva. This time, my heart opened to my own pain. Where did that dolphin get the courage to withstand such pain and fight for her life? It would have been easier for her to die.

Captiva was ultimately pulled through the operation by her connection with Jayne Rodriguez, her closest human friend, who was there comforting her and talking to her throughout the procedure. In one awful moment Captiva's breathing stopped, but Jayne did not let go, repeatedly calling Captiva back to life. Amid the turmoil, confusion, and separation she was experiencing, Captiva's tenuous link to Jayne helped her hear and respond to Jayne's voice. Captiva took another breath. So did I.

Suddenly I knew what I would need to survive further medical treatment: someone who would not turn away from my pain, just one person with an open heart, or perhaps, a dolphin…

I began to understand my dream. Though we reach out in darkness, someone will be there. When I reached out for help, half dead and filled with cancer, dolphins came to me in a dream. It was easier for me to connect with dolphins, whose state of consciousness is akin to unconditional love. Cancer patients and others in search of healing would one day connect with me. *This golden connection heals.* Call it love, the glue of life.

Captiva, unwillingly captured for the entertainment industry, died in the fall of 1989, despite the medical intervention that extended her life. *Captiva, the dolphin, is in my heart.* And now, she lives in yours.

Bernie's Comments

When you let your heart make up your mind and you pay attention to your feelings, you make better decisions. Terri and Amy did just that, in the story "Nameless," when they volunteered to rescue animals and stepped in to save the life of an abused and neglected dog.

Animals live from their hearts more than from their heads. When they are rejected or abused and they don't feel any love, that's when they withdraw and close up. They may fear punishment, but it's the absence of love that's the worst thing in their life.

My mother was in labor for days and too ill to survive a cesarean section. When they finally pulled me out, I was so bruised and swollen from the contractions and the forceps delivery that my mother described me as a purple melon. They didn't know what to do with me except hide me. It would be devastating for a kid to remain hidden and not be touched, and fortunately I didn't have to experience that for long. My grandmother stepped in, pouring oil over my head and body five or six times a day, massaging me and pushing everything back where it belonged. I went from being isolated to feeling like the most loved kid on the planet, because I was massaged every few hours. We now know that infant massage stimulates brain development, weight gain, growth, emotional stability, and more. Those body memories remain stored in us.

Down at the shelter, when the animals run out and embrace you, and you respond to them, this changes the animal. The good part is when they're not afraid to come to you and wake you up to the fact that they are beautiful creatures. When I see an animal curled up in the corner, shut down, I feel that emptiness, and I go to it and pet it to wake it up again. How much your touch means!

In Sandra Pollard's story, "Tokitae," human beings captured animals for their pleasure. Animals don't do that to one another. We need to respect them and care that our actions have long-term, enormous consequences.

The Bible tells us to turn to nature to find answers. In *The Book of Changes*, or *I Ching*, ancient sages used wisdom gained from nature to solve problems and make judgments or prophecies. While putting up a fence in our yard, I nailed the fence to a tree. Over the years I watched the tree grow around the nails and fence. What does that say to me? Here's something irritating, and the tree grows around it. It takes it in; it embraces it. How many people are like that? When a stream hits a rock, you don't hear it yell, "Who put that rock there?" The ocean doesn't complain about the shore. Instead, the sound it makes is beautiful. When we listen to these sounds, we relax. Nature doesn't fight itself; it comes together, forms a unity and completeness.

The ancient dance of the orca: someday we all will dance that dance. It may look a little different on water than it does on land, but it's still the dance of life. When we can all come together, we will free ourselves. And when something we do takes a life, whether we're cutting down a tree to build a house or having a meal, we'll say, "Thank you for your gift." Vegetarians will thank the vegetable for providing them with nourishment, and flesh-eaters will thank the animal. It's the attitude of the person toward all living things that will free all life on the planet. We will provide one another with what is needed, rather than use one another and kill for pleasure — like killing elephants for their tusks, and animals for their fur, and so on.

"They will release me from the sea pen" could be a metaphor about us. We are all confined — although we humans create our own pens. We imprison ourselves by the lives we lead. Only when our lives relate to and harmonize with nature are we not penned in. And whether you're in a hospital room, your place of work, or at home, if you can look out a window and see nature, or if you have photographs and paintings of natural scenes on the wall, then your body experiences less stress. Nature provides that gift. It's our therapist.

In "The Stowaway," as the kitten was bathed and it accepted the warmth of the water, the act became a baptism of love. When we have reverence for life, we express this by our actions, like those of the couple who braved the swearing cat. We change consciousness — ours and others'. We are constantly changing the physical world with our consciousness. When we have a negative attitude — bitter at the world, resentful — it has a negative effect. Healers direct their consciousness in a positive way, helping the world. We can all be healers when we understand this practice and integrate it with our daily lives.

In "Captiva the Dolphin," the dolphin, like other sea

creatures, understood that consciousness is always there. It's not about *who* gets in the water with them; they "hear" people's consciousness, and they know they can communicate with that person or other creature. They don't have to know the person's history or anything else. You could say that Janet, in this story, was playing the dolphin's role. Dolphins are usually teaching us, but in this instance the dolphin became the student.

5

Synchronicity

She [dreamt]...someone had given her a golden scarab. ...While she was still telling me this dream, I heard something behind me gently tapping on the window.... It was a scarabaeid beetle,...whose gold-green color... resembles that of a golden scarab. I handed the beetle to my patient with the words "Here is your scarab." This... broke the ice of her intellectual resistance.

— Jung

When the seemingly perfect timing of two or more events creates a beneficial transformation involving circumstances or understanding, we may be experiencing what Jung called synchronicity. He coined the term. Jung was fascinated by this phenomenon, in which time seems not to exist, events line up or appear to be reset in some divine order, and things happen that cannot be explained.

These perfect connections don't arise from a state of chaos. Instead, they occur when we align with the universe by means of positive, healing, love energy. When we make decisions and choose behaviors that are life *enhancing*, the positive effects of people and things that come into our lives are no coincidence.

I had just written a book about a boy whose dog, Buddy, dies. The boy can't get over his grief, and he has a dream about heaven, where all the dogs who died recently are walking along, holding a candle in one paw. But his dog's candle is unlit. When the boy learns from his dog that no matter how often they light it, the boy's tears keep putting Buddy's candle out, he lets go of his grief and starts doing the things Buddy would want him to do and enjoy. After that, Buddy isn't in the dark anymore, and his spirit can go and do what it needs to do. The book is titled *Buddy's Candle*.

After finishing the book, I took Furphy out for a walk, and I heard a voice say, "Go to the animal shelter." When I arrived at the shelter and opened the door, there was a dog sitting in the corner, looking dejected and sad. I asked, "What's his name?"

"The owner brought him in less than fifteen minutes ago. His name is Buddy."

The rescue center never leaves animals by the door; they're always kept safe in kennels down the hall. This dog had only just been dropped off. If I had arrived just a few minutes sooner or a few minutes later, or if the dog's name had been Spike or Joey, it would have been a different situation. But I came at the perfect time, and he had the perfect name. This was no coincidence. Buddy was *meant* to be there.

"I'll adopt him," I said, because I knew it was meant to be, and Buddy came home with me.

The next stories involve animals that got what they needed because the people in their lives were doing things in response to what they felt in their hearts. They were aligned with the universe. Timing, circumstances, and events together turned these people into makers of miracles — angels in human form.

Facebook Ferdie

ANDREA HURST

~≈~

It was nearing Thanksgiving, and I sat at my computer trying to distract myself by browsing Facebook. The loss of Chloe, my beloved dachshund, was still fresh after four months of heartbreak. We'd been through so much over the eleven years we'd had together, and I felt lost without her. My other dog, Basil, a long-haired doxie, sat all forlorn by the front door. Without his lifetime pack leader, he refused to go for walks; and I worried I'd lose him too.

Each time I visited pet rescue sites searching for another dog to fall in love with, I just didn't feel ready to adopt. I considered fostering dogs through a local dachshund rescue. Posted on their page this day was a fund-raising request for a dachshund's surgery, along with a photograph of an x-ray of the dog's spine. How well I recognized that kind of back issue. Chloe had gone through spinal surgery when she was only four years old. If it hadn't been for the kindness of others who helped pay for her expensive surgery, I would not have had those extra seven years with my sweet girl.

This black-and-tan doxie had been hit by a car and was found on the roadside, lost and starving. Tamara, a kindhearted woman in Southern California, rescued him from the local kill shelter days before he would have been euthanized. His leg was dragging, and his pain was obvious. She brought him to a vet, who suggested immediate surgery to salvage the leg by inserting a pin to hold it. Here on Facebook was the x-ray, along with a plea for donations to help pay for the surgery.

I could help! In Chloe's name, I paid it forward the way others had done for her surgery. Then I posted the dog's story and fund-raising request on my Facebook page, and some of my friends donated. A few days later Tamara posted an update: the surgery had gone well, and the doxie boy was now recuperating. Yay!

A few weeks later, still thinking about fostering, I gave my name to Patricia, a local woman who helps several rescue groups, which range from Southern California all the way to Canada. Besides working a full-time job, she rescues and transports doxies and arranges temporary foster homes for them.

Another month went by and Christmas was approaching. It wouldn't be the same without Chloe's little stocking hanging from the mantle or her sweet, warm body curled next to mine under the down blanket. Basil kept close to me, but he seemed to be fading, as if losing his will to live.

The week before Christmas, Patricia contacted me. A male doxie with health issues was being driven up north along with other rescued dogs. All the dogs had homes waiting in California, Oregon, or Washington, except for this boy, Ferdie. He needed a foster home until after Christmas, when Patricia could take him to a group foster home in Canada. Could I provide temporary fostering?

I asked what his health issues were. She said he'd been hit by a car, had leg surgery, been neutered, had several teeth removed, and would probably need more extractions. He was still on pain medication but recovering well.

"Is he the boy whose x-rays were posted on Facebook?" I asked.

"He is the same dog."

I had given help in Chloe's name; it seemed now she was helping me and saying, "It's meant to be." I told Patricia, "Yes!"

Late the next night, I drove to pick Ferdie up. When I brought him home, Ferdie looked around and immediately wagged his tail. Good start. The next morning after breakfast, Basil and Ferdie got acquainted. Basil seemed interested in the new addition, then settled into his usual spot on the couch and napped. No problems, there.

I took Ferdie onto my lap. He gazed up at me with the most loving eyes I had ever seen. In my head I kept hearing, "It's you, it's you." This went on for hours, both of us just staring at each other in loving recognition. He'd been through so much and still didn't have a forever home waiting.

Within two days I knew that Ferdie and I were meant to be together. There was no way I could say good-bye and pass him to another foster home. I called the rescue people, and to my relief I was allowed to keep him. I'd been told there would be several health issues ahead, and there were: from pancreatitis to bladder crystals, to the need for another surgery on his leg. I was never sure how long Ferdie would be with me, but one thing I did know: I would love him and take care of him as long as he lived.

A few months later, Ferdie needed extensive surgery to remove the pin, which was migrating into his leg muscle. I turned to the rescue people and asked for help in raising funds online. Sure enough, kindly friends and strangers donated generously, and the costly surgery was covered. Good deeds just kept pouring in; even the surgeon, who went beyond what he'd promised to do, did not charge extra.

I'm happy to say Ferdie is still with me, newly nicknamed "Velcro Dog," for he's always in my lap sleeping or performing cute antics that make me laugh. Basil and Ferdie love to go on long walks these days. We're all looking forward to our second Christmas together and hoping for many more to come.

Bacon, Songs, and a Prayer

Lyn Kiernan

❧

I lived under the deck of a drug house with my mom and siblings until I was three months old. Humans threw food over the edge of the deck, and Mom led us out to eat. Then we ran back and hid. We learned from our mom that these humans were to be feared. A few of my siblings got sick and died. No one cared.

One night I heard sirens, loud bangs, and screams. People ran everywhere. Men with sticks and guns surrounded the house. Bright lights flashed. We huddled under the deck, shaking. Suddenly a big light shone on us. Someone said, "Check under there. Looks like animals." They used sticks with wire loops to grab us by our necks and drag us out. I knew about humans — to fear them. They will hurt you.

They took us to a place with loud, barking dogs and locked us in cold cages. Humans looked at us through the wire, calling us over to them. My brothers went, but I was too scared. If anyone tried to pick me up, I would defecate. So no one took me home. I was the most fearful dog anyone had seen at the shelter.

My two brothers bit me. I was the runt. The humans took them away to protect me. Now I was really alone. My brothers got adopted in a week.

A woman came in to put a collar and leash on me. She was patient, but I was terrified. When she touched me

I yelped. After a few more attempts she invited me out of the cage on my first walk ever.

Others came — volunteers — and did the same. I just wanted to get back to my cage and hide in the corner. I did not want to be seen.

At four months of age, I was visited by a human I'd not seen before. She seemed to know about me. She was one of those volunteers. Strangely, she did not try to put me on a leash or touch me. She came often, four days a week, and sat on the floor in my cage, saying my name, Wally, and staying a long time. She talked softly and sang to me, songs only I could hear. I liked that.

After a few of her visits, I wasn't shaking as much. She always brought treats, different from the dry, crunchy dog biscuits. I could never eat them while she was there, or else I would throw them up, but she left them in a little pile next to me. My favorite was the bacon treat. Sometimes she would cry when she left.

"I want to adopt you and pay for an animal behaviorist to help you overcome your fears," she said. I didn't understand her words, but I listened to her feelings.

"But they have regulations and laws here. My fence at home is five feet high. For your breed, it has to be six." I heard the frustration in her tone. The next time she spoke, another feeling came from her heart and entered mine.

"But don't worry, I won't give up trying."

She didn't give up.

At seven months of age, I was still not adopted. My friend came to tell me she could not visit any longer.

Heartbroken, and with no hope of helping me, she had to stop fighting the system. She cried a long time and turned her back to the open cage door so people could not see her.

I let her touch me that day, let her rub my legs and massage my ears and neck. I did not shake, and we were both shocked. It didn't hurt at all. She said a prayer for me, saying it was the most powerful thing she could do.

One day I got adopted by a human who had heard my sad story. I went home with this stranger in a car and hid on the floor, curled in a ball. Their house had an older female that did not like me; she bullied and bit me. This was my first experience in a house. The man of the house really scared me, and I ran from room to room to get away from him. He was only trying to be a friend, but I didn't know that. One day he got too close, too fast, and I barked at him. They called the shelter. I was going back.

That's when the miracle happened. Someone at the shelter had heard the singing human's prayer and seen her crying. This friend put the two households in touch by phone, explaining if I were returned to the shelter there would be no hope for me. So they had to bypass the system.

Now I was in the car again, curled in a ball on the floor with all my things, but this time they took me to another strange place and led me down a path. Nothing looked or smelled familiar.

That's when I heard a voice call my name — Wally. I knew that voice. As we headed toward it, I smelled bacon. It was my singing human. I pulled harder, moving faster and faster to get to her. I was overjoyed to see her. I must have eaten a pound of bacon that afternoon!

I'm four years old now, and I live with humans who love and understand me. My best friend and playmate, Murray, taught me everything I needed to learn about being a dog. We are the same age, both from the house of cages. Murray and I have made many friends, both canine and human. These people are loving, kind, and understanding.

My singing human also dances. I jump around her feet. When she is happy, I am happy. She is still the only one I let hold and kiss me. I go to her all the time for petting. Whenever I'm running free at dog parks with Murray, I return to my human often and check in. I never want to lose her again.

Two-Day Zoey

CARI L. SADLER

She came into our twenty-four-hour veterinary hospital as a found stray. During ten years of working there I had, through my unaffiliated rescue group, taken in so many strays and owner-surrenders that the Tampa hospital's euthanasia rate was lowered. I can honestly say each animal touched my heart, but Zoey and her story stand out as exceptional.

She was a two-year-old, red shepherd mix with a microchip. Even an unregistered microchip gave me some ability to follow a trail. Zoey's chip had been implanted by the high-kill, local Animal Services Department, and they provided me with the last-known owner's contact information. As Zoey sat quietly next to me, the owner's voice on the phone said, "We don't want her."

I looked down at her big brown eyes and whispered a promise: "Don't worry; you're *not* going back to death row."

When I contacted one of my foster families, they gladly offered to take her in. My rescue organization, Cari's Keepers, consisted of vet technicians, a few local veterinarians, and volunteers who fostered the animals. I was blessed with a good reputation and a well-organized network.

Two days after placing Zoey in the home, I received a phone call. "We're sorry," said the volunteer who had been fostering Zoey, "but you have to come get her. She does not know anything. She's not housebroken. She doesn't even understand the word *no*. She's like a wild child."

I went and picked her up. Zoey was excited to see me. I called a rescuer friend who had her own foster program. After hearing the circumstances, she offered to take Zoey under her care. Given the hour-long drive, I bought a plain hamburger for Zoey and me to share along the way. She licked my hand gratefully and then rested her head against me.

Two days later my phone rang: "I'm really sorry, but she needs more one-on-one training than we can handle. You'll have to come and get her."

Once again Zoey was excited to see me. I scrambled to think of what our next stop would be. On the drive back, a lady I had not previously worked with, but who came with good references, called. She said her own dog had been exactly the same as Zoey when first taken in, and that she would gladly take Zoey into her home and work with her. After driving two hours we finally arrived. The lady was standing outside with her dog and with expectations of instant bonding. What was instantly apparent to me was that this wasn't going to work. Back in the car we went.

Driving back to our starting point, I called my hospital's owner to inquire if weekend boarding was possible. It was a long shot, since it was an emergency/specialty hospital and not set up for boarding.

"If I do it for you, I have to do it for everybody," he said.

I began to panic. I was running out of options. Then the rain came, and it rained hard. With Zoey next to me, I began to cry. Was I really going to have to euthanize this beautifully tempered girl because of my lack of resources? I drove, and for the first time in a long time, I prayed.

I called my husband, who listened while I vented. He suggested I contact a local animal hospital, update needed vaccines, and board her for the weekend to give me time to figure it out.

A girl named Shallie answered the phone. "We definitely have room for her," she told me. "I'm also going to give you my dad's cell phone number. He's been training dogs in Tampa for forty years."

After Zoey's appointment and boarding arrangements were settled, I called Clarke, Shallie's dad. "Bring her to me Monday morning so I can evaluate her," he said. Finally she was in a safe place for the weekend, and I had a glimmer of hope.

Monday morning Zoey was excited to see me, and we drove to Clarke's training facility. Taking her leash, he instructed me to sit quietly while he assessed her. Within *five* minutes she was doing *everything* he asked her to do! I apologized for the tears streaming down my face. He smiled and then offered to train her at no cost, put her in his adoption program, and find her a forever home. Clarke's program requires every member of an adopting family to attend each training session, giving animals the highest chance of a successful forever-home outcome.

It wasn't until days later that I learned Shallie, who doesn't work the phones, *just happened* to be at the front desk the day my call came in. I also learned that several veterinary specialists I work with had used Clarke's services for their own pets.

Had any part of this rescue gone differently, from the intricate timing of events to the people who were involved, Zoey's story would have ended with a devastatingly sad good-bye. Upon reflection I realized I was never the one steering my car or her rescue. Was it divine intervention? What about my prayer for help? With much gratitude I now realize both her life and my heart were truly saved.

Miracles on Demand

CINDY HURN*

~⚬~

In my profession as a life coach and hypnotherapist, I also teach personal development classes. On one particular winter's evening, I had been talking about the power of positive thinking and how we can affect one another just by the way we choose to communicate. When we use negative comments and focus on what is wrong with the world, the energy of that exchange supports negativity and fear. The world energetically darkens. But when we choose to focus on the positive and share with others from a lighter and brighter perspective, the energy uplifts and enlightens them. A positive focus is a simple way not only to help ourselves feel better but also to beneficially affect those around us.

I went on to introduce miracles, explaining that they come in all shapes and sizes and occur all around us, but they can easily go unnoticed. Sharing a few miracles that had happened to me, I asked my students to be aware of how they felt after hearing the miracle stories. The lesson of the last miracle was that we can either open ourselves to hope and possibility or wrap ourselves in limited thinking.

Inside the classroom, a slumbering butterfly had awoken despite it being the dead of winter. Throughout

---

* The story contributor Cindy Hurn is not the same person as Cynthia J. Hurn, Bernie's coauthor of *Love, Animals & Miracles*. See the "Story Contributors" section at the back of the book for further details.

my lecture this beautiful winged creature was fluttering about in the zigzag flight pattern typical of butterflies.

At the end of class I gave a homework assignment that would amplify the lesson and encourage awareness during the week. Reminding my students that miracles come in all shapes and sizes, big and small, I asked everyone to be open to a miracle happening during the week and come prepared to share its wonders with the group the following week. I emphasized the importance of not judging their miracle, for judgment diminishes the experience. The second part of the assignment was for everyone to tell another person about their miracle and observe what happened to the listener.

Throughout my delivery of this homework assignment, my butterfly friend had continued its fluttering pattern, lightly dancing around the room. Ending the class, I stood up with both arms outstretched and said, "Now go and find that miracle!"

At that moment the butterfly stopped zigzagging and flew in a straight line across the large room, directly at me. With perfect timing, on the last word of my sentence, it landed on my forehead, right on my third eye. Our eyes met just before it landed, and when it settled above my brows I felt this delicious energy flow through me. I had been kissed by a butterfly!

With such sweet grace my winged friend had provided perfect material for the second part of the homework — a miracle for my students to share with others.

Bernie's Comments

Andrea Hurst's story, "Facebook Ferdie," is a wonderful example of synchronicity created by our consciousness. When this dog is on her lap, looking at her, he's communicating. It's only when Andrea is willing to quiet her mind — not thinking, "What should I do; can I handle this?" — that the dog can communicate to her, letting her know she's the one. We can also see in the interconnected events of Ferdie's story that when you're making life-enhancing choices for everyone involved, the act of giving comes full circle. The one gift inspires another, and that gift brings about the next, so the giving has no end, like an eternal circle of love.

The story "Bacon, Songs, and a Prayer" teaches us that when we are quiet, we get our true reflection. When Lyn came to volunteer, she didn't think, "I'm here to walk a dog." All the other volunteers tried to drag the dog out for a walk, but Lyn stilled herself and paid attention to the dog's signals, listening to what *he* needed. She sat with him, gave him treats, and sang; she calmed the frantic energy; she became his still pond.

Not only did she respond to the dog in the way he needed, but she also was open to asking for help — she prayed — and her prayers were heard, or in this instance overheard, by the person who intervened and became God's instrument. Each event — including the dog's initial adoption, which got him out of the rescue center in the first place — worked in synchronicity, creating perfect harmony for the last stanza of Wally's happy song.

"Two-Day Zoey" exemplifies these words from the Bible: "I have set before you: life and death, blessing and curse. Therefore choose life" (Deuteronomy 30:19). What we find with Cari and all these people is that their choices and activities made the difference. Divine intervention isn't God looking down and saying, "Okay, let's be nice there"; it's *you* making the divine intervention. The forces of nature and creation are available to all of us, and we are the battery cables. We deliver the energy. We become a blessing — God with skin on.

A stricken animal can be healed of a physical ailment or emotional behavior, or it can be rescued from a difficult circumstance, but it's our acting as a conduit of this energy and our *desire* to do something that make us all capable of inducing miracles. You don't have to go and find a healer. We are all healers. It's a matter of quieting the mind, believing, and making the effort.

"Miracles on Demand" reminds me of a lecture I gave in Hawaii, where a butterfly became my helper. I wrote about it in my book *The Art of Healing*. In that experience, I talked to the creature like it was a member of the family. I said to it, "Okay, this is what we're going to do. I'm going to put you in a bag; I'll take you to my lecture, and when we talk about the symbolism of the butterfly and transformation, I'll let you out." The butterfly, whom we had rescued in unusual circumstances, chose to remain with us for two days and had no problem going into the bag, sitting there, and not feeling confined. It was a mystical experience.

Butterflies represent the soul and spirit in us, which makes me wonder if the butterfly in Cindy's story was connected to her through some person in her life — manifesting that person's spirit — by giving her a kiss and being with her. *How we think* induces these connections and miracles. You can just as easily block them from happening if you're creating a negative field. So, if you want to attract miracles for those you care about, open your heart, still your mind, and listen.

6

Animals Who Serve

Tiger's temperament is as soft as his body. When I see
him, it knocks the chaos of war down several notches.
He's my little piece of sanity...makes us laugh and raises
our spirits in this desolate, harsh place...Afghanistan.

— Staff Sergeant Jessie Walker

At Amsterdam airport, when personal items are discovered in the terminal or abandoned on the plane,
an enthusiastic new member of the airline's lost-and-
found team is dispatched. Today Sherlock is wearing his
bright blue vest with wide pockets on either side. When
he's told that a treasured item is still on the plane, he
races, all on his own, to the arrival gate and jumps aboard
the aircraft. A crew member produces a soft toy bunny
and Sherlock studies it with his nose. The attendant puts
the bunny into Sherlock's vest pocket, and then, off he
goes! With ears flapping like hankies in the wind and tail

alert and wagging, the specially trained beagle follows the scent of the lost object's owner. Sherlock navigates long walkways, leaps over piles of luggage, rides the escalator down to the baggage claim, and follows the scent till he finds the owner. A little girl has been crying for her lost friend, and she looks up in surprise when the beagle gallops up to her, stops at her feet, and sits. Her delighted parents remove "Barney the Bunny" from Sherlock's pocket as the canine hero receives a grateful hug from the girl. With one more mission successfully accomplished, Sherlock returns to headquarters for a biscuit.

When animals are trained to utilize their naturally endowed gifts, they can do remarkable things to serve humans or other animals. The key to their success is that they are doing what they love to do, and they are rewarded with generous measures of food, play, and affection.

Neuroimaging studies of dogs' brains have revealed that when the animals look at their humans, as opposed to a stranger, the reward pathways of the dogs' brains are flooded with oxytocin, the bonding hormone that is also released in mothers when they hold or nurse their infant child. As the researcher Brian Hare puts it, "When your dog is looking at you, he's hugging you with his eyes." Studies also reveal that when human beings look at their dog, the brain wave changes are identical.

Some animals intuitively provide valuable services with limited or no training. My dogs Buddy and Furphy come to all my cancer-support-group meetings. Buddy is intuitive and senses people's health status. He'll walk up to somebody who's talking, and he'll look back at me to say, "This guy is doing well." When he finds people who aren't doing so well, he'll go and give them some love, not looking to be petted, but just to rub against their legs and give them healing love and attention during the group meeting. Furphy, on the other hand, is self-centered. He retreats under my chair and takes a nap. They know that when I give them a treat it means: "Okay we're starting now." Furphy lies down and goes to sleep while Buddy does his rounds.

One man arrived a bit late on his first day in the group. He sat down and started sharing all the tragic events related to his cancer. Suddenly the sound of snoring filled the room. The man became really upset, saying, "What's wrong with you people? I'm telling you about my life-threatening illness, and you're falling asleep!" Everybody was waving a hand and pointing under my chair, where Furphy was curled up snoring. That turned out to be the most therapeutic thing that happened for the man that day. He looked under my chair and then burst out laughing.

Another time, Furphy came with me when I was giving a lecture at a university. As I stood before the audience and began to speak, Furphy howled, ran onto the stage, and jumped up against my legs, yapping. I felt terrible. Here I was, trying to give a lecture; people couldn't hear me, and I was apologizing like crazy while not knowing what was wrong. Then I realized that although a few hundred people were in attendance instead of half a dozen in a group, to Furphy it was still a group. I told people he was saying that I forgot to give him a treat. A man ran out of the building and came back with a biscuit. I gave it to Furphy, who then walked off the stage, went over to the corner, and fell asleep. Everybody burst out laughing. Furphy was giving us all therapy. The next stories involve animals who, trained or not, gave service and saved lives in many different ways.

A Princess and a Duke

BARBARA J. HOLLACE

⧂⧂

During the time my husband and I ran a homeless shelter for people, we had a dog named Duke. He served as guardian and protector for us and for children, his special love. Duke was a golden retriever–chow mix with the sensitivity and loving nature of a golden and the lionhearted-defender spirit of a chow — an ideal match for us and the people we served. He became a hero to those who were victims or who had no voice.

There was one special child who would arrive at the office door and ring the bell every morning, eager to make the same request for much-needed company. One day Taylor's shoulder-length hair was dirty and disheveled, and more than likely she had missed breakfast. Maybe her mom was having a rough day and her dad had gone to work.

Opening the door with a smile, I greeted her, "Good morning, Taylor."

"Can Duke come out and play?" she asked.

"Sure. Duke can come out. Would you like a snack?"

Normally we didn't offer food to our residents, but this little one was an exception to the rule. Taylor hesitated. Likely she had been told not to ask for food, but she was seriously hungry. It was a tough decision to make. Finally, without saying a word, Taylor nodded her head. Technically she hadn't asked for food.

"Okay, I'll be right down with Duke and a little snack." I left her waiting outside the front door. We never invited anyone upstairs to our apartment; everything was done in plain view.

I made a peanut butter sandwich, having discovered on one of our afternoon walks that it was her favorite. Liberally applying the peanut butter, I also gave a generous helping of tender loving care. Duke danced around my feet; he knew who was waiting for him downstairs. He loved this little girl with an extra measure of love, if that was possible. Somehow he understood that her home life wasn't so great. Dogs and children go together like peanut butter and jelly, and the friendship between these two proved it.

I put him on his leash, and down the stairs we went. I'm not sure who had the biggest smile when we approached the front door, Duke or Taylor. On most days that Taylor came to visit, we would either take a walk or weed the green space in the center of the parking lot. Today we stopped for a little chat on the curb while she ate her sandwich. Duke was attentive to every crumb that dropped, but refrained from asking for a bite. Taylor needed it more.

Duke loved her simply by being there. She offered him love in return — the love she so badly wanted and desperately needed to receive. Theirs was a relationship at soul level, and they communicated using a language of the heart.

The happy ending to this story is that several years later my husband saw Taylor with her new family — a relative who had taken her in. "She looked like a princess," he said. "She's blossomed into a beautiful flower of a girl."

If Duke could speak, I know he would say that this princess flower was part of his handiwork. Love seeds, once planted, bear fruit. It may take time, but unconditional love never falls short. If you don't believe me, ask the princess, Taylor, and Duke, her knight in shining fur.

Surf Lifeguard

❧

Bilbo, a Newfoundland dog, first visited the lifeguard depot when he was fourteen weeks old. He belonged to the coastal services manager, who often left him with me. We soon developed a strong bond, playing hide-and-seek in the extensive building. When Bilbo reached one year, his owner erected a fence around their house and left him there outside, mostly alone, for the next year.

I had occasion to visit them when Bilbo was two. As I approached their garden, I whistled our special hide-and-seek call. Bilbo instantly remembered me and tried without success to scale the fence. Part of my job involved inspecting all the emergency telephones and lifesaving equipment stationed on coastline footpaths. I told his owners that Bilbo could accompany me for these occasional daylong walks. I'd return him to his home at the end of each inspection day. On one occasion circumstances demanded that we go out for three uninterrupted days. I returned Bilbo to his home that Friday; on Sunday his owners phoned to say he'd kept them awake all night, howling. He'd also gone off his food. How did I feel about taking him on full time? I agreed on one condition: he had to have permission to be with me in the office during winter and on the beach in summer. They agreed, and that's how Bilbo's career in lifesaving began. He would never be left on his own again.

The first few months with Bilbo were difficult, to say the least. At two years he was almost fully grown, weighing 196 pounds. From nose to tail he measured five feet, seven inches, and from head to floor, thirty-six inches. I lived on the cliffs above the beach where I worked. My house was a small shed that had been converted to living quarters with basic necessities. Every time I rose from a chair, Bilbo, determined not to be left alone again, would spring up, knocking everything over with one giant sweep of his tail.

One time the wind blew all day from my neighbor's direction, carrying the scent of his female dog in heat. Bilbo grew agitated. Knowing he was agile enough to jump through the window and capable of opening doors, I screwed the window shut and bolted the door securely before going to bed. At dawn, my telephone rang.

"Steve, your dog is in the garden."

"He can't be," I said groggily, but got up to check. That's when I found — like in a cartoon — the Bilbo-shaped hole in the kitchen door and splinters of wood scattered outside.

I soon observed that anytime we went near the sea, Bilbo would get between the water and whoever was approaching it. Realizing he'd be an asset to our lifeguard service, I started taking him along whenever we were doing swim-training routines. Initially Bilbo was apprehensive about the bigger waves, but the bond between us was so strong that he'd follow me anywhere. Soon he was taking on head-high breakers.

Newfoundland dog teams demonstrate rescues wearing harnesses with handle straps on the back. A dog swims to the person in the water, who grabs the handle, and the dog tows them back to shore. In reality, anyone fearful of drowning would certainly *not* look for a handle but would simply climb onto the first thing that appeared. They could easily drown a dog.

I trained Bilbo to use a Peterson tube instead, a standard piece of the surf-lifeguard kit. This flexible float is attached to the rescuer by a two-meter line. Bilbo was trained to swim *around* the person in the water, avoiding their grasp while drawing the tube close enough for them to grab. Once Bilbo could feel tension in the line, he would tow the casualty ashore.

For five years Bilbo worked alongside our professional surf lifeguard team on Sennen Beach, near Land's End, Cornwall, England, and he saved lives in many ways.

Many people disregard the signs that direct beach-goers to "swim between the lifeguard's flags," and they won't even talk with us if we try to explain why the flags are there. But Bilbo was a social icebreaker between lifeguard and public, making our jobs much easier. When people saw this bear-sized dog wearing the yellow-and-red lifeguard's jacket, they'd come over to meet him and talk to us. We'd explain the dangers of undertow currents or of swimming too close to the granite cliffs, where waves could smash them against the rocks. Suddenly their attitude about heeding our advice changed. Once their respect for the lifeguard was established, the number of incidents involving unsafe actions on the beach dropped remarkably.

Bilbo can sense if a situation is good or bad. He's trained to bark when he sees an arm waving in the water and respond only at my signal, but on more than one occasion he's picked up on a bad situation and dispatched himself to deal with it.

People don't realize that ocean waves come in sets, with each wave in the set being of similar size, and that every once in a while a substantially bigger set will come crashing in. Parents think their kids are safely playing in knee-deep water, but it may, all of a sudden, rush up to their chests and stay chest deep for possibly six or seven waves. Adults who aren't vigilantly watching, or who aren't close enough to respond quickly, risk losing those children. It takes only an instant. One day some children were in such a situation. I walked over to the parents to advise them of the danger, but Bilbo wasn't prepared to wait. He wanted those children to be safe *now*. He went straight to the kids and barked until they got out of the water.

Another time, sea conditions had changed dramatically from the day before, producing much bigger waves and a strong undertow. I'd been checking emergency equipment at a remote cove, when a woman trotted down the cliff path. "You're not planning to go into the water, are you?" I asked her.

"Yes! I swim every day we are here," the visitor responded in a foreign accent.

"It's not safe today; I wouldn't go in if I were you," I said as she passed. A minute later Bilbo made one woof, alerting me to look back. The woman had laid out her towel and was now heading straight for the sea.

Without prompting, Bilbo charged down the cliff, onto the beach, and planted himself between her and the water. When she tried to go forward, he stood on her feet and barked. Waving her arms, she yelled for me to call my dog off, then pushed past Bilbo and headed toward the water again. He dove into the surf, trying to block her. It wasn't until she saw Bilbo struggling against such powerful waves that she realized how strong the current was. She admitted afterward that he'd been trying to communicate with her and that she hadn't listened.

I have no idea how many lives Bilbo has saved or who they were. Most were holidaymakers who came and vanished back home again. Recently a young woman visitor approached me in town, saying, "You don't remember me, do you?" I didn't and admitted so.

"Bilbo rescued me down at Sennen," she said. "Nobody realized I was in trouble. He swam over and stayed by me; then he towed me back to shore."

In 2009 Bilbo was invited to Crufts in London, the world's largest dog show. He was awarded "Dog of the Day" in the working dogs category, and the following year he was made "Pet Hero of the Year."

After Bilbo retired from lifeguard duty, he began spreading his beach-safety message at schools. Although I do the talking, the kids look at Bilbo as I explain the danger of digging and climbing into deep holes in wet sand. Teachers are amazed how long kids sit still, totally absorbed by Bilbo's tranquil, majestic aura.

For this retired surf lifeguard, the most remarkable thing about Bilbo is the unbreakable bond he formed with me eleven years ago. When that playful chocolate puppy walked into the depot, he changed both of our lives for good.

Read between the Paws

JENNY PAVLOVIC

❧

A little girl jumps up and down when Chase enters the library. She read a story to Chase last month and wants to read to him again. She doesn't have a dog at home. With his back legs and rump up, Chase bows down and hugs the floor with his elbows, lowering his muzzle so it's not in the girl's face. He is repeating the same polite "let's play" greeting that he instinctively adopted on the first day he met this nervous child. She claps her hands.

"Look, Mommy, he's bowing!"

Chase remains calm while she keeps jumping with excitement. And when she settles down on the quilt, he snuggles in next to her and gives her his undivided attention as she reads a story to him.

Just learning to read, the girl easily becomes frustrated by new words. She's also been teased and bullied on the playground at school. I want to build her confidence, to let her know how beautiful and smart and wonderful she is, and to show her that encountering something unfamiliar, such as a new word, can be like discovering a treasure.

Our library visits were originally about helping kids learn to read. But Chase and I found we can also be an antidote to bullying, offering true friendship that cushions her in a world that sometimes feels unkind. Fifteen minutes of friendship and undivided attention not only

120

builds the girl's confidence in reading but also makes a positive difference in her self-esteem. All the while, she is learning to love and be kind to dogs.

Chase is highly intuitive; he knows exactly what she needs. I realize that he knows just what I need too. He led me into this work. I sometimes wonder who's getting the most from our visits: the little girl, Chase, or me. Fifteen minutes pass quickly, and another child is waiting with book in hand. It's time to say good-bye until our next session. During the month between visits, I often think of the little girl, and I look for books that she might like to read. I wonder if Chase thinks about her too.

I call my mom, a teacher — now retired — who specialized in reading. I ask how to help the child with her stumbling blocks and frustration. I'm amazed at how much my mom knows and am grateful that she instilled in me a love of reading, a love for books so deep that I not only read them but write them too. This brings me closer to Mom. I don't have children of my own, but I remember sitting in Mom's lap while she read stories to me and, eventually, I read stories to her. At the library I've learned that I too love listening to kids read.

Chase came into my life after Hurricane Katrina. I had gone to Louisiana as a volunteer to care for rescued animals. If not for our common mission to help displaced animals who were lost in the hurricane, I never would have met Sarah, another volunteer, who lives a thousand miles from me. Sarah rescues animals in a poor area of rural Virginia. She listed a red heeler mix on her website after rescuing him from an angry man who threw him around, stuffed him into a tiny chicken crate, and was planning to shoot him for chasing sheep. When Sarah went to get him, the dog sat on her lap and shook for a couple of hours despite her soothing assurances that now he was safe and no one would ever abuse him again.

Sarah and I determined that this dog would likely be compatible with my Australian cattle dog, Bandit. With the adoption arranged, he then needed transport from Virginia to Wisconsin. Volunteer relay drivers stepped up to the plate, and a friend of Sarah's in Indiana put him up for a night while he was en route. I met the dog in Wisconsin and brought him home to Minnesota. He earned his new name — Chase — because that's what he most loved to play with Bandit.

Chase and Bandit were soon best buddies. In spite of coming from a violent and troubled past, all Chase *ever* had to give was love. His gentle nature and affection for people led us into meaningful, life-changing work. After we earned the therapy dog certification, we joined the reading program at the local library.

Surely it wasn't just chance that brought Chase into our lives, but a series of everyday miracles sprinkled along the path to Bandit and me. It seems this wonderful teacher in a fur coat was born to help children develop reading skills and to teach all of us about love. So many insignificant events led to that magical moment when Chase made his first bow to the nervous child and, in her delight, she lost her fear and began to jump up and down. If *dog* is truly *God* spelled backward, I think that was the day God winked at me.

Maltese Miracle

Ruth Vanden Bosch

≈

Bernie Siegel and I have done many workshops together. We met while I was recovering from surgery. Like most people who have had cancer, I worried that it might return. I knew one thing for certain: if I didn't stop my old lifestyle of caring for the world, I would get sick again. But helping people was my profession and a great part of my life. There had to be a way to love the world and help those in need without sacrificing my health! I prayed, asking for guidance.

When the flyer came in the mail — a holistic psychology course that featured Dr. Bernie Siegel and several other holistic practitioners — I knew it was God's answer. Many of the conference speakers were survivors who spoke eloquently about how to live a healthy life after cancer. They'd made major life changes, such as giving up smoking, becoming a vegetarian, and exercising daily. I appreciate the value of a healthy lifestyle, but I needed something more; I was seeking an inner peace that didn't include worrying about the possibility of the cancer returning.

Bernie's lecture helped me the most. He talked about being able to say no when you don't want to do something. This would be a struggle for me, as a registered nurse and a psychologist, to adopt. I rarely said no to any request and found it almost impossible to stop trying to please everyone. Bernie helped me understand that my personality was programmed long ago by my family. As a perfectionist, people pleaser, and success junkie, I could not accept failure in myself. Being a preacher's kid, I'd always had to be the perfect example for other kids. "Don't forget, everyone is watching your behavior!" still shrilled from its tenured perch on my shoulder.

Listening to Bernie and reading his books, I realized I could rebirth myself as a new person and stop trying to please everyone. It is okay to just be me and to have faults. My past thinking was driven by a need for the acceptance and love of *others*, but my new awareness gave me freedom to love myself and parent myself. What a revelation!

Another change occurred in my life at this time. My friend Shannon raises teacup Maltese show dogs. The demanding criteria for show dogs include perfect physical characteristics of the breed. Two of the Maltese criteria are a flawless black nose and black markings around each eye. All of Shannon's puppies qualified, except for the runt of the litter. The black circle went only halfway around his left eye; and because his trachea collapses whenever he is excited, he honks like a goose! No one wanted the imperfect puppy. For love of myself, I adopted the puppy; and to honor Bernie Siegel, I named the puppy Bernie.

Perfectionism was killing me, but breaking the habits of a lifetime is difficult. Little Bernie became the answer to my prayer. His imperfections don't worry him, and he doesn't care about mine. He simply loves me. Bernie is my constant reminder that it's okay to let go. I can make mistakes; I am forgiven and loved anyway.

If I'm ever upset or depressed, Bernie hops onto my chair, plants his tiny body next to mine, and lets me know that he is right by my side. If anyone tries to move him, he growls his displeasure and refuses to leave me. He listens when I tell him my problems. He looks at me as if to say, "Breathe — everything is happening exactly as it should."

One day a man came to spray ants that were invading our condominiums. I had just had knee surgery and was lying on the couch with my right leg elevated on pillows. My knee was wrapped in elastic bandages and a knee immobilizer. When the man came into my condo, Bernie sensed something about him that he didn't trust. Bernie stood on top of me, growled, and bared his teeth. I suggested to the man that he do his job and leave; and with Bernie's encouragement, that's exactly what he did. The next day, I learned that the same man had attempted to rape my neighbor. Bernie had given no thought to his own safety. That man could easily have injured or killed him. The fact that Bernie weighed only four pounds was not an issue. He accepted himself as he was and thought only about his job — to love me and protect me from danger.

Bernie is now a therapy dog and frequently comes with me to visit my patients when they are hospitalized. Being so small, he can fit into my purse. My patients and counseling clients adore him. He looks into their eyes like he is saying, "Lean back into the arms of grace. Let go and let God."

Am I more content because of a Maltese named

Bernie? Oh yes. My little angel — my personal miracle — reminds me every day that I am everything I was ever meant to be. It's okay if people consider me to be a bit of a character, and it's just fine to say no. Last of all, he assures me that I don't have to grow up. That could be bad for my health!

Bernie's Comments

Barbara's story, "A Princess and a Duke," shows an animal's capability to give friendship so willingly. Duke knew who was waiting outside and understood the child's needs. He was reading the girl's consciousness, actually feeling what the girl was experiencing. When speaking from heart to heart, you don't need words. Compassion is felt; you don't have to say anything. When Barbara gave the girl peanut butter sandwiches, she responded to one of the girl's hungers. But it wasn't only her act that fed this child. The dog was giving her love; that's what Taylor really needed.

In "Surf Lifeguard," Steve and Bilbo show that the bond we form with animals often surpasses that which we have with people. Animals' minds are quiet. Because they are open to us and possess that state of acceptance, we know they're not judging us. It's similar to Furphy whining when he wants to go out; it's not personal, he's not evaluating me; he is just expressing his desire to go out.

Steve mentioned the challenges he faced with Bilbo. If we could treat one another the way we treat our animals, we'd have much happier relationships. It's not about the two people in the relationship; it's about *creating that third entity*. Bobbie called it a struggle being married to me. Joseph Campbell referred to marriage as an ordeal. What they are saying is that you have to work at it. It isn't just the needs and wants of the individuals, or of the person and the animal; your ordeal is about creating something new, a relationship where $1 + 1 = 3$, the third entity.

People are more forgiving of their animals than of other people. For example, when our dogs poop and pee in the house I don't curse at them or throw them out; I simply go and clean up, because I know there's a reason it happened. We are less tolerant of our children and spouses. Instead, when they do something we dislike, we ask, "How can you behave like that? What are you doing?" We're always analyzing and judging; we think too much. Animals are not; they are feeling.

When you listen to your feelings and let your heart make up your mind, you live a very different life. Steve and Bilbo weren't thinking only of themselves. They were going out there together and making a difference. The *entity of love that was created between dog and human* was what became the lifeguard, saving others and themselves.

Jenny and Chase offer more than one gift in "Read between the Paws." When I've taken my dogs to elementary schools, afterward there was always at least one kid who'd say, "I was afraid of dogs, but I'm not anymore." I'd be reading a story with the kids sitting on the floor; each dog would walk over to a child and sit on the child's lap — nothing else, just sit there. The dogs seemed to know which kids needed love most. Kids learn then that dogs will be there for you, with you. In the animals' presence they don't feel like victims.

I'm reminded of a magnetic car sticker in the shape

of a paw. It says, "Who rescues whom?" Dogs also help us enjoy being in the moment. A plaque in my mother's home said, "Enjoy yourself; it's later than you think." I don't remember seeing this plaque in all the decades my parents lived in that house. But when we went to clean the house after my mother's death, there it was on the den wall as you entered; you couldn't miss it. She'd hung it there before she died. It would be her last message. Now it hangs in my house.

Ruth has the nurse personality, always trying to fix everything, do everything, as she explains in "Maltese Miracle." Nurses have a hard time saying no, and they don't take care of themselves. But dogs follow their hearts; this dog is a wonderful teacher for her. He became her therapist.

Trying to live up to some image or idea leaves you feeling inadequate. We are perfectly imperfect. We have to accept that about ourselves. If you feel good about yourself, you're not worrying about being normal or perfect. Furphy has been attacked by other dogs. He's lost an eye and his tail, but that doesn't stop him from appearing in public. He doesn't focus on it. Dogs know to just be their authentic selves.

Animals can be intuitive about humans or about another animal. Ruth's dog, Bernie, wasn't analyzing the stranger who came into her condo. He acted on his own intuition, alerting Ruth that the man was suspicious, and this made the man uncomfortable.

When I first adopted Furphy, I was traveling a lot, and I didn't like being out there alone all the time. He'd stay in hotels with me, and he would growl when some-body went by in the hallway — letting them know: "You'd better not come in here." I got such a kick to know that a little guy like him was protecting me.

What Ruth didn't mention was that her friends know that she knows me, so when she talks about Bernie, they think she means Dr. Siegel. Soon after she got the dog, somebody came to her door and heard her yelling, "Bernie, get down! Get off me! Stop doing that, Bernie!" The person at the door, thinking it was me in there, didn't know what to do. Should they go away, come back and ring the bell, or what? When Ruth heard a noise at the door, she opened it, and the visitor was so embarrassed; it was hysterical. Ruth told her about the new dog, and they had a good laugh.

7

Paw Professors

The great pleasure of a dog is that you may make a fool of yourself with him and not only will he not scold you, but he will make a fool of himself too.

— Samuel Butler

There's a story about a man who goes to a zoo where the animals live in designated areas protected by fences. He mistakenly enters the tiger's area and realizes he is in danger only when one of the tigers starts coming toward him. He runs to the edge of a precipice, grabs a vine, and climbs down to where the tiger can't reach him. He thinks, "Okay, I'll go all the way down and find my way out." But as he's descending, he sees another tiger looking up at him. He thinks, "Now what am I going to do?" Noticing some wild grapes growing on the vine, he picks one and eats it. "Ahhhhh." The message of this story is: you may have a tiger in your future and a tiger in your past, but eat the grape and enjoy the moment!

Animals don't lecture us about what we've done wrong. They show us by their behavior how to be and how not to be. We often teach them useless things, like "play dead" or "shake a paw," because it's cute, while the things animals teach us are valuable — things about loving and living. When you can be as good as your dog, you have accomplished a great deal.

In the next stories, five grateful students share lessons they learned from their paw professors.

Shifting the Energy

C. M. BARRETT

⚶

Many years ago I had an encounter with a cougar, which has stayed with me ever since. Despite my ambivalence about going to places where wild animals are held captive, friends of mine persuaded me to go to a wildlife farm.

Soon after we arrived, we came upon an enormous, mighty cougar pacing back and forth in a small cage. I stood, shocked and helpless, wishing I'd never agreed to come. Overwhelmed with pity, I felt the burden of this beautiful, and now powerless, creature inside those steel bars. How could we do this to wild animals? The cougar paced, his eyes avoiding my pitying stare.

After a few moments I realized that my reaction to the cougar's reality certainly wasn't making me happy, and I could do nothing to change his circumstances. More important, was my attitude doing the cougar any good? I believe animals are aware of our thoughts and emotions, and mine were incredibly bleak at this point.

The only thing I could change was me. How could I shift my reaction? The answer came to me the instant I asked the question. I looked at the magnificent cat.

"You are so beautiful," I said, as my heart overflowed in gratitude. "You are so powerful. I love you. Thank you for your presence." The big cat continued his pacing. Was it my imagination, or did I see him glance at me as I walked away from his cage?

Half an hour later, I passed the cat's cage again, and this time the animal greeted me with that unique cougar screech. I paused, and it screeched again with greater urgency. I stopped, turned back, and walked closer to its cage. The majestic cat looked into my eyes, rolled over on its back, and purred.

Tears blurred my vision. As I write this, they reappear, and I cherish that memory. He taught me there is always something I can do, always *something* I can add to any situation, no matter how sad or unfair. When I sent love and gratitude to the cougar, the burden he carried was momentarily made lighter. For that one moment there was no cage, not even a cougar and a human, just two beings joined in appreciation and the spirit of love.

Love Lessons

Darlene Cloud

≈

Although I'm not a novice dog owner or guardian, I have learned so much from our golden retriever. Cuddles arrived at the Homeward Bound Golden Retriever Sanctuary in Elverta, California, with no hip joints. Unable to walk, she dragged herself by her front legs and was in constant pain. Homeward Bound arranged for her to have a total hip-replacement surgery.

Ralph and I adopted Cuddles when she was only six months of age, two weeks into her recovery. The first surgery was not successful, owing to her faulty bone structure. Over time Cuddles had to endure a total of four hip surgeries and months of rehabilitation. Nevertheless she awoke each day with a look in her eyes that said she was ready to take it all on.

Lesson learned: Each day is new. Take it as it comes.

At five years of age, Cuddles is still making up for the time when she was unable to run and play. She is the happiest of dogs and loves everything! Carrots and her dog food share top billing as her number one love, people are a close second, and third are her toys.

Lesson learned: Don't dwell on the past; enjoy what you have.

She is patient. I have to admit, patience is not a trait I normally associate with dogs. Her patience wins out over mine when it's close to her dinnertime. She will sit beside her bowl and proceed to stare at me, barely blinking. That stare gets to me, and don't think she doesn't know it!

Lesson learned: Think positively, and things will go your way.

Cuddles lives up to her name. Wherever we are, there she is. At the dinner table, she's by our feet. On the couch, she's in my lap, all fifty-three pounds of her. In the kitchen, we are stepping over her. Why not make her move, you ask? Just look at her face and you'll understand. She must be close to us — that's just her. Cuddles also lies on my side of the bed each night, much to my husband's chagrin as he struggles not to fall off his side. He really is an understanding man.

Lesson learned: If you know who you love, stay close by.

Although small for a golden retriever, Cuddles has a way of making her presence known — for example, her nose in your face if she thinks you have slept enough, or her head in your lap if she thinks you've been on the computer too long. She brings one of her toys and drops it at your feet with a loud *kerplunk* if she thinks it's about time you got up and moved.

Lesson learned: Take time to play and have fun.

Each day, as life brings lows along with the highs, it's a blessing to have Cuddles to teach me by example how to love and to enjoy the moment. It's a tough lesson for humans to learn at times, but I've got a great teacher.

Morris the Cat

GLORIA WENDROFF

≈

For two years Morris came and went. My daughter, Lauren, thought he was a stray cat gone wild who had probably been on his own for most of his life. Lauren owned a house on an acre of land with hundreds of trees and berry bushes. We lived there in adjoining apartments. Lauren's side of the house had three outside doors, while I had one front door and an inside door connecting our apartments.

Whenever stray cats came to one of my daughter's doors, she took them in and kept them or found them homes. There were so many! But Morris dared only to come near Lauren's door after she left food outside and went back in, closed the door, and remained out of sight.

Unbelievably, about six months after Morris first appeared at Lauren's door, he started to appear at my door instead. You have to know that all my life I'd had a cat phobia. Cats terrified me so much that I had recurrent nightmares about a cat jumping from a tall staircase and landing on the back of my neck.

Well, there he was, alone and hungry. I started putting food out for him. Each time, he would run away and return after I'd gone back inside. Morris, the cat who was so afraid of people, was coming to the door of the person who was so afraid of cats.

A friendship grew between us. After several months,

I could bring myself to pet him, and he brought himself to let me. At some point, he learned to trust me enough that he would come into my front hall for a few seconds, then panic and run out. I started to leave the front door wide open so he could escape. We tamed each other.

Little by little, Morris began to stay inside for longer periods of time and allow me more physical contact through petting and stroking. Then one day he accepted my house as his home, but only when *he* wanted to come in. Morris was still a free agent, coming and going as he pleased, yet he was my cat. During the nights he always stayed out.

One evening I was standing on a chair to change a lightbulb in the bathroom. I fell onto the edge of the bathtub, broke seven ribs, and had to stay in the hospital for ten days. During this time my daughter never saw Morris, not even once.

The morning I came home from the hospital, there was Morris, sitting on the front path waiting for me. Still in pain, I couldn't climb the stairs, so I slept on the couch.

Morris no longer went out at night. He slept in the house. *Morris slept in the house!* He curled up on the chair across from me and kept an eye on me all night, every night. He watched me in the day as well.

In about a month, I was able to go upstairs and sleep in my bed. Each night, Morris wanted to come in and sleep with me, but I wouldn't let him. We'd have a race for the bedroom door, and each time I "won." It was a great disappointment to him, and the resigned Morris slept outside my door. I had always let dogs sleep with me, but never cats. I wouldn't sleep with a cat. Somehow, I just couldn't let the idea go.

On the night that turned out to be the last time Morris would try to get into my room, he almost made it into my bedroom before I closed the door on him. But this time, instead of sleeping outside my door, as he had every night before, Morris went downstairs and howled at the interior door to Lauren's apartment. Lauren let him in, and, for the first time, he slept with her. She was happy to have him. How I have wished since that I too had been happy to have him. I would be so happy now.

That was the last night Morris would be refused entry into my room. It was the last time we ever saw him. He was gone — simply gone. We never knew what happened to him.

I have wondered if Morris was an angel, his mission to be responsible for me. Maybe he'd been granted only a certain length of time to be with me, hence his need to sleep in the same room. And I wouldn't let him. There are many times when I think of how hard he tried to enter my bedroom, and I want to apologize to my feline friend, saying, "Oh, how I want you, Morris, the blessing of you."

Now I try to honor what only he could teach me. I pick up cats and hold them on my lap, giving them the love and comfort they need and deserve. Morris overcame his fear of human company and touch; he showed that when we accept each other with unconditional love, there is no room left for fear.

Italian Lessons

Ali Le-Mar

Mole came to us three years ago, aged seven weeks, an adorable little bundle with knowing, humanlike eyes. He is a special breed of dog called Italian spinone, sometimes referred to as Italian griffon. With long, droopy ears, a full beard, and a mustache, he looks like a comical, pipe-smoking old duke. Mole approaches the world with a laid-back attitude, meaning he does everything in his own time and his own way. But don't let that fool you; his muscular seventy-pound body is a testament to two thousand years' worth of hunting-dog genes.

What we initially thought was stupidity and stubbornness turned out to be intelligence and sagacity. At gundog training, our other dog will go like a bat out of hell, in a dead-straight line, through thick, prickly undergrowth to retrieve the object. Mole, on the other hand, will assess the situation and work out the best way to go around obstacles, regardless of how long it takes. Mole thinks deeply about things and how to carry out tasks. When everyone assumes he's just goofing off or confused, or has lost the scent altogether, he suddenly gets the job done.

Mole also goes to agility classes — in fact, he's become an agility superstar, once again proving everybody wrong. No one expected such a big, lumbering dog to be so quick and agile. Our Mole is full of surprises!

We compete all over the country at field archery

events, and our dogs come too. Wherever we go, people stop us, wanting to meet him and ask about him. Sometimes it gets a bit crazy as we travel only a few yards before the next person stops us. They usually talk to him before they talk to us. We have been fortunate to meet some lovely people through Mole!

Earlier this year Mole began to limp, favoring one leg, and we could find no obvious cause. Rest didn't improve the situation, so we took him to the vet for further testing. I received the devastating news when my other half was away attending a seminar: Mole had an incurable bone cancer, painful and extremely rare in a dog of his youthful age. I called my partner, and he came home right away. Our world seemed to collapse as we faced Mole's terrible prognosis. We prepared to say good-bye to our dear sweet friend.

The vet wasn't prepared, however, to give up on Mole. He persuaded us to have his leg amputated, saying that we had to give him that chance. We didn't want to put Mole through any further pain, but the vet reassured us that he would soon heal, and the pain would be minimal. We agreed to go ahead.

It was an exhausting, emotional time for us, second-guessing our decision. Would Mole ever again be able to do any of the things he loved? Would this operation just prolong a painful disease that might kill him anyway? What would the quality of his life be?

Word spread about Mole's condition. Messages of love and support came to us from people all around the country — many of them virtual strangers to us, but all of them people who had met and fallen in love with Mole. In only three years Mole had touched the hearts of many. It wasn't until then that we realized the impact this thoughtful dog had had on people. Their concern and well wishes for Mole's recovery was astonishing, and it really helped us through a difficult time.

Two days after surgery the vet brought him home to us, a bit wobbly and bewildered. After one week Mole was getting around pretty well on three legs. After two weeks his stitches were removed, and he could go on short walks. Three weeks later, Mole was zooming around like he always did. Now he's back at gundog training, still doing things his way, but most important, still doing things!

I feel utterly humble in his presence. Throughout the events of these last weeks, Mole has acted with enormous courage and immense dignity; not once has he whined or made a fuss. Mole has taught me so much — how to chill out and be patient is the greatest lesson. Watching him endure this ordeal and maintain a serene outlook makes me realize that I've got nothing to moan about. If he can overcome this, then I too can overcome anything thrown my way.

We don't know what the future holds for our noble, majestic Mole. We may have him with us for only six more months, or we may be blessed with six more years, but the important thing is that we still have him, and we will ensure that the rest of his life is as action packed and fun as his first three years. No doubt Mole will continue to surprise us and teach us in his quiet, laid-back style that no matter what happens, life really is worth living to the utmost.

Bernie's Comments

In "Shifting the Energy," it's only when C. M. Barrett recognizes the cougar as whole that they both find a sense of peace. What a beautiful memory. And what a powerful effect it has, because the cat knew what this person was thinking and gave her what she needed. When she learned that she could look at the cat, see his beauty and power, and say "I love you," he knew it was true. He could feel her sorrow and know that she cared. The cat knew she wasn't the one who did this to him, and so he could give her that love and help her feel better. It was no longer about him being a captive but about mutual love and respect — a gift. Just because you're in a cage doesn't stop you from giving something to others.

Reading "Love Lessons," I smiled at the image of the dog's nose thrust into the writer's face. Our cats do this with their tongues. Cat tongues are really rough; it's like waking up to sandpaper rubbed on your face. I pull the sheet over my mouth and nose, and the cats know: not tonight; you don't get to do that tonight. Animals are trying to be affectionate, but sometimes, ugh! My cats and I do head-butt kisses instead.

Animals' patience is so important, and even more so is their willingness to listen to you. When people start giving you advice, you may not get anything out of it, or you may not be ready for the solution. But when the animals listen, you hear yourself. You're more likely to pay attention to yourself and your feelings when you're talking to an animal, because you're not having a dialogue. Often when you are teaching or coaching others, you end up hearing what you needed to learn.

"Morris the Cat" shows how fear creates a barrier to love. Morris felt the opposite of love — rejection — and so he left. I'd say to Gloria, "Send him your thoughts of love and sorrow, and he might return. Send him a thought message with your thanks every day, telling him you love him and would like to have him visit." If he's still around, I bet he'll come back. Not only do animals teach us to forgive others, but they also teach us to forgive ourselves.

"Italian Lessons" reminds me of one of our rescued buddies, a wirehaired pointing griffon mix. The griffons have kind, humanlike eyes. We went down to adopt a dog at the shelter. One of them jumped up and gave me a bloody nose, but we adopted him and our son took him home. Another one that we rescued would run around while on a leash, tie everybody's legs up, and knock them over. Bobbie named him Bruiser — really appropriate. Everybody who met these dogs loved them; they were real characters.

I knew someone whose cat was in the hospital, and the vet called to say their cat wasn't going to make it. He suggested it should be euthanized. So my friend said, "I'm coming in; I'd like to be there with him." The whole family drove over to the hospital in tears. The vet brought their cat into the examination room, carrying the little creature in his hands. But when the cat saw the family, it jumped out of the vet's hands, flew about eight feet across the room, and landed on its owner's chest.

"He was dying an hour ago," the surprised vet said. They told me this story two years after the incident, and the cat was still going strong. So there's another lesson in this: When you're sick, be among those you love. Even if it doesn't cure you, you'll exceed expectations. Ali's dog can feel his family's love, and so he's happy. He has everything he wants. He doesn't think he's missing anything.

8

Sometimes They Just Know

If a dog will not come to you after he has looked you
in the face, you ought to go home and examine your
conscience.

— Woodrow Wilson

A woman I knew was riding through familiar territory with a group of friends when her horse came
to a sudden halt and, despite all urging, refused to move
forward. My friend had a deep bond with this horse, and
so she knew something was wrong but couldn't see what.

"Kitty always leads the others because of her steady,
bombproof nature," my friend said, "but this time one of
the other riders had to take the lead, hoping Kitty would
follow. It didn't work; Kitty still refused to budge."

Seconds later, the horse and rider who *had* gone
ahead disappeared in a cloud of dust. The earth had literally swallowed them up. Luckily, the horse managed to

climb out of the sinkhole without losing his rider or suffering any injury.

So how did Kitty know what was lurking ahead when the other horse didn't? Was the special bond between Kitty and her rider a factor? It's possible. Animal intuition is often heightened when it involves a close relationship. One man told me he couldn't get his dog to leave his sick father's bedside. The dog would go in the kitchen only to eat, and outside only to pee and poop; the rest of the time he stayed in the father's bedroom. One day this man found the dog in the kitchen. He said, "I knew my dad was better, or the dog wouldn't have left him. I went into Dad's room, and sure enough, he was on the mend, showing signs of improvement."

Our cat Miracle used to sleep on my chest whenever I was unwell. I didn't ask her to; she came because *she knew*. When I was feeling good and just having a nap, she'd be playing outside. The following stories illustrate just how intuitive animals can be, whether it's about someone they love and who's cared for them or someone they hardly know.

More Than a Lab

The local pound had a limited budget and an unlimited supply of residents. As soon as the black Lab–golden retriever puppies began eating soft food on their own, they were put up for adoption. The pups were only five and a half weeks of age. We picked one from the litter and agreed to return for him the next morning after all the documentation had been approved.

The next day my son had to go and get the puppy for me, because I had hurt my back and couldn't make the drive. He came home with a pup from the same litter, but not the one we'd originally chosen. When I told my son, his face dropped and he offered to take him back and get the right dog.

"There is a reason for everything," I said. "When a greater hand than ours intervenes, I think we're being shown that this puppy is meant for us." And so began our journey with Boo.

He grew…and grew…and grew even more. Boo didn't stop growing when he reached the size of a Lab, nor that of a golden retriever. He kept gaining height, length, width, and weight until he was bigger than any dog I'd ever owned. It turned out that our Boo was a black Lab/Irish wolfhound mix.

Nobody told me what to expect from a wolfhound, especially the noise that would emanate from his throat when he started baying at the door. At first we had no idea what was wrong when Boo released a sound like a roaring windstorm playing the long notes of a dirge.

"Oh, woe, woe, wooooaaahh," he sang, as his lament filled the whole house. What I wouldn't give to hear that baying one more time.

Boo was a bit of a handful. At one point, whenever anyone said good-bye he'd become upset. He would block the door. He would growl. Once he even snapped at a girl my son was dating. She thought it was cute to make him growl when she said good-bye, and she pushed her luck. Not wanting to take any chances, we called a dog behaviorist. This man showed up wearing a long trench coat and carrying a brief case, looking more like the exorcist than a behaviorist. But his modifications to *our* behavior were certainly effective on Boo's.

"No bones. Nothing is free. He is not your baby. Treat him like a dog." I never could figure out what that last directive meant, and yet, in spite of all the things we did right or wrong, Boo turned out to be the perfect dog.

One day Boo began barking like a crazed animal at the front window, which faces our neighbor's house. I looked to see what he was trying to alert us to, but nothing out of the ordinary was apparent. No matter what I said or did, he wouldn't stop. Finally, just to quiet him down, I took him over to the neighbor's. It turned out that my elderly neighbor had fallen and landed on top of her cat. The cat was biting her, but the woman was unable to get up off the cat. We helped her up and released the angry feline, and Boo was declared a hero.

Boo lived to a ripe old age. When he died, we had him cremated, intending to bury his ashes in a beautiful spot. But his ashes are still on my bureau along with his picture; I just can't seem to let him get too far away from me. The exorcist was wrong about one thing: Boo *was* my baby!

Raising the Alarm

R. Ira Harris

My son, Max, at thirteen, had never ridden his bike beyond the flat streets of Sacramento, California. One afternoon I packed Max, his bike, and Sammi, our year-old Australian kelpie, into the SUV and drove to visit my cousin Ken, who lives on a mountain near Napa Valley.

Ken's house is situated at the top of a mile-long gravel driveway, and while we were there, Max had a great time racing his bike down the drive. After visiting for a few hours, I started to pack the car for our return to Sacramento while Ken and his family left for some event they were attending. As soon as the car was ready, Sammi hopped in the car and took up her position in the back seat. But Max pleaded for one more descent.

"Okay," I said and followed him in the SUV. Knowing this was his last ride of the day, Max raced down the hill as fast as he could, but this time he lost control. The crash was not a pretty sight. I scooped up Max, put him in the car, and sped back up to Ken's house.

Leaving Sammi in the back seat, I took Max inside. Bits of gravel had gouged his skin, and blood streamed from the wounds. As I comforted him, I wondered where Ken kept his first aid kit, and that's when the car horn started to blare. I ran downstairs to find Sammi in the front seat, pushing on the car horn with her front paws.

"No!" I said, rebuking her, and returned to Max. The

minute I reentered the house, the horn sounded again and then stopped. It was only a few moments later when several neighbors, including a nurse, burst into the house. That nurse was a godsend.

"How did you know I needed help?" I asked.

Ken's neighbor explained that in their community, where people's homes are a bit isolated, they had formed emergency response signals. A repeated horn blast is a cry for help.

I figured that Sammi must have sounded the horn by accident the first time and possibly did it again out of curiosity or boredom. She had never done it before. But now that she knew how, I expected her to try the horn whenever she was left alone in the car. That wasn't the case. Never again did Sammi sound the horn.

Sammi's instinct that day was to raise an alarm for a wounded member of her pack. But how did she know that the horn, rather than barking — her natural noise-maker — would bring help? Maybe I will never under-stand it, but one thing I cannot deny is that her action has bound us magically together forever.

Diag-nosed by Dog

Alyson B. Miller-Greenfield

❧

We had three rescued Labs at our home in Colorado. Dakota was black, Dillon was yellow, and Baci was a dark chocolate brown. Each one came to us with a sad story and little eccentricities. Dakota and Dilly were the elders, and they generously took it upon themselves to initiate Baci, the newbie, into the culture of our pack.

There came a time when Baci would not leave Dilly's head alone. He started licking him, and kept on licking the same spot for several days. No matter what I said to dissuade him, Baci seemed determined to lick some invisible thing away from Dilly's fur. Finally I said to my husband, "Maybe Baci knows something we don't."

I took Dilly to the vets' office. They could find nothing wrong during the examination, but when I told them about our other dog's insistence on licking the spot, they decided to investigate further. Tests revealed a cancerous growth under the cartilage of Dilly's ear where it joined his head. This growth was completely invisible to the human eye! Stunned and delighted, we called our chocolate hero Dr. Baci from then on. He literally diagnosed the cancer, and he did it just in time to extend Dilly's life.

Dilly and Dakota have long since departed and crossed Rainbow Bridge. Now Dr. Baci is fourteen and is having his own health problems. But the other day a friend, who, unbeknownst to us, had taken a tumble earlier that morning, came over for a visit. As soon as our friend arrived, Baci went directly to him and started licking his knee. It seems that as long as he is with us, our doctor dog will never retire.

Feral No More

RITA CELONE UMILE

≈

My mom once rescued a cat so wild that only when she left food in an isolated place would the cat appear at all. Any chance of people being in the vicinity would send this cat scampering. Mom was determined to domesticate the wild thing before our cold Connecticut winter settled in, so she remained consistent in her feeding pattern regardless of the animal's shyness. She named the cat Nina.

After several months Nina learned to trust Mom, but only to the point of entering the house for food and nighttime shelter. Nina was not in the least affectionate: as soon as her meal was finished she'd retreat and hide, her seclusion undisturbed, until morning, when she went out again. Mom came to expect little companionship from this feral feline.

Then one day Mom took a tumble down the cellar stairs. Although not seriously injured, she sensed that her ankle had been more than twisted. The intensity of the pain indicated a fracture. It was late in the evening, and she simply did not have the energy to take herself to the emergency room. Instead she took to bed, whimpering in pain.

Lo and behold, Nina emerged from her nightly hiding place, jumped on the bed, crawled under the covers, and wrapped herself around Mom's broken ankle. How did she know? Mom was amazed and grateful. Nina stayed in this position all night, gently licking Mom's ankle, an incredible sign of sympathy and an attempt to give comfort. Nina and Mom, from that night forward, have remained bonded as only the best of friends can. Mom's patience and respect for Nina broke through this wild creature's reserve, showing her it was okay to trust. Nina's newfound ability to express her love was born of one thing: my mother's persistent, selfless acts of love.

Bernie's Comments

"More Than a Lab" may seem remarkable to us, but it must have been unbelievable to Boo that his humans didn't notice somebody was in trouble, that they weren't responding. What was wrong with them? No wonder he made such a racket. Our dog Buddy makes so much noise that we don't need a doorbell. No thief could sneak into our house. Floss wisely said that a greater hand than theirs chose the dog. If we all responded to so-called mistakes like she did — not blaming the person for bringing home the wrong dog, not making a big fuss — we'd make room for more miracles in our lives.

"Raising the Alarm" brings to mind how my wife, Bobbie, responds when people ask, "Where did that come from?" She says, "It came from God-knows-where." That's the only answer. How did the dog know the horn would bring help? That knowledge came from God-knows-where. Yes, the neighborhood consciousness focused on taking care of one another, but it takes a dog to be quiet enough to connect with it. Sammi wasn't in a panic, thinking, "What can I do?" She was connecting with the consciousness and responding intuitively by putting her paws on the horn. This is what life was meant to be like. Animals understand, and live according to that understanding, every day, while we're thinking and struggling, not living the message. And when Ira says it "bound us magically together forever," I say, "Bound together, yes;

but it's not magic. It's *real*. Intuitive love was built into us by our creator."

"Diag-nosed by Dog" is a great example of people being open and not going around saying, "That's crazy, and I can't accept it because I can't explain it." The vets didn't try to *explain* what the dog sensed or how he sensed it; they accepted that it happened and responded appropriately. If you open your mind to possibility, you learn from it; you become wiser and better educated. Refusing to accept something just because you don't understand it is like rejecting a gift. Things aren't there for us to judge; they're there for us to use and learn from, so why not be grateful and accept the gift? Tell Baci that I said, from one doctor to another, "Nice work, Dr. Baci. Good boy."

Rita's story, "Feral No More," exemplifies how love benefits both the giver and the receiver. When someone is upset, breathe in their anger, their bitterness, and trouble; then exhale love toward them. That's what animals instinctively do. They take your pain and then give you love and compassion to replace it. How often we sit down after a hard day, stressed by life's demands; our dog comes up, puts a paw on our laps, and gives us a look of understanding; or the cat curls around our stress-knotted shoulders and starts purring, giving us a massage.

Doctors need to learn from animals to be compassionate. If you treat the disease but not the cause, you're not helping people. Animals instinctively treat the cause.

9

Miracle Healers

Without your wound, where would your power be? It is your melancholy that makes your low voice tremble into the hearts of men; the very angels themselves cannot persuade the wretched and blundering children on earth as can one human being broken on the wheels of living. In Love's service, only wounded soldiers can serve.

— Thornton Wilder

Animals, through their own wounds, recognize the troubled human being, and they create a relationship. They don't judge; they pour love and acceptance upon our wounds. They understand.

When a group of people gather to work on a project, to learn something, or to take up a creative endeavor, you have the makings of something inspiring — something transformational. Too often we find reason to judge others, and to project our problems onto them, thereby diminishing ourselves and one another. But when we become like the animals, when we encourage one another and allow a space where exploration and respectful, nonjudgmental feedback can happen, it changes the way we see ourselves and others. We become students as well as teachers. We grow on many levels. We become greater parts of the whole. And this, I'm certain, is what life is supposed to be about. Little steps combined beget great journeys.

Some of the following stories involve people gathering for just such a purpose — to explore, to learn, to celebrate. During these gatherings, individual miracles happen. In the other stories the lesson is the same — one of connection — and through this connection, a greater awareness is born and new life begins. These stories are about healing and growth. They are about unlocking and changing states of mind that hold us back, and about the animals that accompany us through the portal from ordinary to extraordinary. They show that when our minds and hearts are open, we truly become purveyors of the divine. We are all miracle workers.

Saber-Toothed Healer

CINDY HURN

≈◊≈

In April 2014 my husband and I traveled to Brazil to partake in a Native American ceremony called the Sun-Moon Dance. This four-day ceremony originated from the vision of Beautiful Painted Arrow, a Ute-Pueblo medicine man.

The dancers go without food and water for the duration of the ceremony. Dancing to and from a single tree placed in the center of a large arbor, they commit to reviewing their life paths and invite spiritual transition and vision. This was my husband's thirteenth dance, and I was there to support him and the dance in any way needed.

From São Paulo, we set out for the hills and traveled for five hours. Our destination was situated at four thousand feet amid beautiful trees in a cascading, lush landscape against the higher mountains. Upon our arrival, I started to feel nauseous and had a headache, and the symptoms dramatically worsened over the next two days. It could have been altitude sickness, but it wasn't unusual for me to have a strong physical reaction such as this to ceremony.

On the third night, I was unable to stand. I sought refuge in my spacious tent, pitched at the far edge of the camping area. There I lay down and tried to sleep off the intense headache. I needed to relieve myself every twenty minutes or so and did this just outside my tent, because

I was too ill to go any farther. It was annoying having to unzip and zip the tent three to four times every hour, so I decided to leave the door completely open. It made life easier, as well as quieter, for me in my sensitive state.

In the early hours of the night, I awakened and turned over to see a large wildcat a few inches from my face. The magnificent creature was looking down on me with its mouth open and enormous fangs exposed. For a still and quiet moment we held each other's gaze. I did not feel threatened in any way, and I calmly said to the cat, "I can fear you or I can love you. I choose love." I beamed him some love, and he pulled back, sitting on his haunches. I then turned over and went back to sleep. My last thought was "How nice — I get to sleep with a cat."

The next morning I woke feeling really well and full of energy. I told the others about my vision, describing the animal as a saber-toothed tiger or big cat, and said how grateful I was that the spirit came to me and healed me. Shortly afterward, I learned that my vision was not a vision but a reality.

The jaguar had been seen in the early hours of the night just below my tent. I had thought it was a saber-toothed tiger, a species now extinct, for when I turned over, those teeth were so close to my face they looked huge. It was explained to me that the jaguar, a large Brazilian wildcat, kills by piercing the back of its prey's skull with its canines.

On returning home I became aware for the first time of the numerous images of jaguars I had previously placed around my house, a few of them my own drawings.

I guess we know more at one level than we realize. My relationship to this animal, once found on the outer edges of my consciousness, now takes center stage.

Since the nocturnal visit of that magnificent jaguar, many things in my physical life and spirit have shifted; a knowledge previously hidden deep within me has woken. I now understand that the saber-toothed healer will always be part of me. I share this deeply personal story only because of the powerful lesson I was given. I learned, in that instant, that choosing love rather than fear goes a long way toward changing outcomes; in this instance it saved my life.

No matter what happens, we always have a choice. Choosing love removes the illusion of separation and supports trust. Love *is* stronger than fear.

The Sparrow's Gift

NICK HURN

A few years back an elderly acupuncture client of mine rescued two baby sparrows, and she successfully hand-reared the pair. On the day it was time for the fledglings to fly, the male sparrow flew off and ended up living in the garden and surrounding area. Often when the woman was sitting at the bus stop, the male sparrow would show up, and they would have a chat. But the female sparrow chose to continue living in the house with the woman.

For many years my client had suffered with severe leg ulcers; no treatment had been found that would make them heal. In order to protect the wounded skin, both legs had to be kept bandaged. One day while the woman sat in her chair, the female sparrow alighted on the bandages and started picking at the fabric. The bird continued to do this for several days running, until the woman thought to unwrap the bandages. From then on her feathered friend would alight on her legs each day and pick at the infected skin, cleaning the wounds.

The woman's legs started to heal. When she went back to see her doctors, they were baffled. How was it that this stubborn ailment was suddenly healed? The ulcers were gone, and the skin was now healthy. Smiling to herself, my client said nothing, leaving the doctors to wonder.

An amazing act by this feathered healer happened on the bird's last day. The sparrow flew over to a tabletop where a small red rose had fallen. Picking up the rose with her beak, the bird flew to the woman and — in a final gesture — dropped the rose into the woman's lap. A moment later the little sparrow collapsed and died.

My client's care for the sparrows had resulted in friendship and near miraculous healing, but there was no doubt in her mind and heart that the most wonderful gift of all was that tiny red rose, the bird's undeniable expression of love.

The Divine Within

MICHELE JANE

≈

I was a student of Klaus Ferdinand Hempfling, one of the world's most talented horsemen, at his school and farm in Denmark. His goal is to help students find their authentic beings and to communicate clearly and genuinely with the horse. Using his lifetime of experience and his strong connection with horses, he guided us to see, through a spiritual lens, the relationship that exists between human and equine. As Klaus interacted with the horse, he related his philosophy and methods of approach that resulted in communication with the animal. Watching him work was a riveting experience for all of us, all except one.

This student was a high-maintenance individual who sought attention and disregarded the precise momentum that the classes required. She kept interrupting Klaus with questions unrelated to what he was doing, and she often redirected his attention. The lessons felt somewhat disjointed and occasionally lost their momentum altogether. I found this student extremely annoying and had to control my urge to snap at her.

Klaus's students are given the opportunity to bring their own horse by prior arrangement, and one day the annoying student brought her mare. When class began, the woman and her mare were already standing inside the square pen known as a *picadero*. Klaus uses this adaptable, smaller structure so that horses can run free and choose to follow, or not, the intention of their human partner.

Since we had all attended several sessions, learning Klaus's methods of equine communication, everyone was shocked at the way this woman communicated with her horse. The poor animal cantered around the outer edges of the pen while the owner stood in the middle and swung a rope at her! The horse was frightened by this, and the woman was becoming increasingly frustrated. Klaus stood outside the pen, directly in front of me, watching the ugly performance.

"This might surprise you," he said to the class after observing for some time, "but I am not going to put my hands into that energy."

"What?" I was thinking. "You can't leave it like that!" As if hearing my thoughts, Klaus spun around and faced me.

"Michele, I am going to ask you and two others to go into the arena."

Klaus chose two more women, the youngest in our group and one of the eldest, with me being somewhere in the middle. He called us together.

"What you are going to do," he said, "is enter the picadero and get the lady onto her horse and riding it around."

"Are you insane?" I thought.

This woman had not been on her horse in six years, and right now it was doing everything it could to escape her, including kicking out.

Klaus's quiet but powerful energy demands respect. You just don't question him; you do as he says. Despite my misgivings about his plan, something more was happening inside me: I wanted to help the woman's horse.

Klaus delivered our only instructions: "If you need to

speak, raise your hand, and then all of you come out of the arena. When you have spoken, you can go back in and continue." The observers grew silent, the gate opened, and three students walked into the arena.

As I stepped through the gate, it seemed as if I'd entered a different world. Everything outside that fence and every thought in my mind, except what we'd been told to do, no longer existed; there was only one reality — do what had to be done.

Across the arena stood the woman who had been the source of my annoyance, but now she seemed a different person. All I saw was a little girl asking for help. I walked toward her and opened my arms. She came to me, and I put my arms around her. She cried and I held her for as long as she needed.

When her sobs subsided, I took her hand and walked to the middle of the arena, where her mare was standing. The younger student stood in front of the mare holding the rope, while the older one stood on the other side of the horse.

I placed the owner's hand on her horse's neck and drew her hand down, showing her that I wanted her to stroke the horse. When I let go of her hand, she began to pat the mare's neck with a firm, slapping motion. I shook my head "no" and once again placed the woman's hand on her horse's neck, gently stroking it in a downward fashion. As soon as I let go, she started patting again! This time I placed the back of her hand on her horse's neck. She looked at me and smiled, then began to gently stroke her horse.

Finally the woman understood. Wrapping her arms around her horse she began to weep. I took a few steps back, allowing her to be at one with the animal. It was only a few moments before the woman looked at me, nodded her head, and offered me her foot. Supporting her ankle with my hand, I gave the woman a leg up and she seated herself on the mare. Once again she leaned into her horse's neck and wept. We students remained still, each on a different side of the mare.

When the rider sat up again, the girl standing in front took up the slack of the rope, asking the mare to move forward, but the horse refused. I looked at the girl and held out my palm, asking for the rope, which she placed in my hand. I passed the rope over the mare's neck, tied the end underneath her halter, then offered the improvised rein to her rider. The three of us on the ground stepped back, making room so the woman could ask her horse to move forward — but we remained close enough to act as support. The mare moved beautifully, without hesitation, carrying her rider wherever she asked to go. No saddle, no bridle, just the two of them — and a new way of being.

This experience became my teacher, showing me what I now call "the Shift," the moment a person goes from human nature to divine nature. The miracle that Klaus knew was there, one that stems from love, happened that day. It happened not just to the woman rider but to each one of us in that arena. The healing, on so many levels, was only just beginning.

Targeted by Dolphins

JENNY PAVLOVIC

꧁꧂

The dolphins torpedoed toward me at full speed. With no other option, I had to trust they wouldn't slam into my body. My insides buzzed with tingling vibrations, sonar signals that dolphins use to seek and understand creatures and objects in the water. It felt like a whirlpool bath with strong jets of bubbles aimed directly at my middle. My midsection vibrated as the dolphins swam closer and closer. At the last possible second these marine missiles veered downward and passed just beneath my body.

It was my first time in Bimini, about forty miles southeast of Fort Lauderdale, Florida. I had come to swim with wild dolphins. Mary Getten, my animal communicator friend, led the trip; she'd been urging me to go for years. I'd never been to the Bahamas before, nor had I previously jumped from a boat into the open ocean.

On my first day I panicked after plunging into the sea, and I swallowed salt water when learning to snorkel. The water was clear all the way to the bottom — a depth of twenty to thirty feet. Later that day, I felt nauseous and vomited several times. I'd never been seasick before and attributed my nausea to swallowing salt water and to a poorly timed trip belowdecks while the boat was moving. After vomiting I felt much better. It wasn't until weeks later that I understood what had truly occurred.

Each day in Bimini we swam with wild dolphins. Although I often heard the clicking of their echolocations in the water, I felt that strong buzzing sensation only on the first day. Since that had been my first time in the water with dolphins, I didn't know what to expect. I thought the buzzing feeling was something that happened anytime dolphins approach humans. After swimming with the dolphins for several days, though, I realized the targeted treatment of the first day was unique and *intentional*.

Months before my trip, I'd had surgery to remove tumors from my abdomen. The tumors were benign but painful. One of them had felt like a bowling ball wedged between my kidney and spine. Since the surgery, I hadn't recovered my previous abdominal strength. In certain circumstances, like when lifting something or sitting up from a reclining position, my abdominal muscles would seize up uncontrollably. When this happened I had to lie on my back on the floor and wait till the muscles relaxed again. I couldn't release them myself. Although I was still highly active, I had learned to limit certain activities in order to avoid the uncontrollable and excruciating contractions.

The first time in Bimini when I attempted to slip into the water from the boat, my muscles warned that this position could bring on the dreaded abdominal seizure. I held back, waited until the others entered the ocean, and then took my time going in. But after I was "sonar-ed" by the dolphins, I had no further problem entering the water.

I had read books by Horace Dobbs and others about dolphins healing people physically, mentally, and spiritually. As a biomedical engineer, I know ultrasound is used to treat swelling, and vibration to accelerate bone healing. I hadn't thought about seeking healing when I went to Bimini, but it was obvious that something significant and powerful had happened.

I believe that when I first entered the water, the dolphins sensed that I had scar tissue from surgery or just that I was seriously nauseous that day. Perhaps their intent was to break down the scar tissue, and vomiting resulted as a purging effect. Somehow they knew I was hurting inside, and the sonar treatment they administered healed my abdomen.

When I returned home, I tried lifting heavy objects and sitting up from a reclining position — and suffered no repercussions. My previous limits no longer existed! In a swimming pool, I treaded water, did the crawl, and even tried underwater flip turns, something I hadn't done for years. Flip turns require quickly pulling the legs into a tucked position while rotating the body; then pushing the tucked legs against the pool wall to propel the body forward. This action uses abdominal muscles and would have caused spasms before. In fact, I wouldn't have even tried it. But now I was swimming and playing for over an hour, pushing my limits without one painful contraction!

Swimming in the sea, too, made me feel stronger again. Now I seek more opportunities to swim, something I've always loved to do. In the water I feel closer to the dolphins, even at home in Minnesota, many miles from the sea. I swim without concern about spasms, and swimming helps strengthen my core.

Before this happened, I believed in the *possibility* that dolphins can heal people. But my own magical experience showed me that it's true. These beautiful creatures of the sea really do have the desire and the ability to heal others.

Bernie's Comments

"Saber-Toothed Healer" brings to mind Carl Sandburg's poem "Wilderness," where he writes, "I got a zoo, I got a menagerie, inside my ribs, under my bony head....I am the keeper of the zoo."

Who is in charge of this menagerie inside of you? You are. The jaguar inside of Cindy spoke to the cat in the tent: "Let us choose love." Love affects the other animal, and the whole menagerie quiets down. Even animal trainers teach us that when we're walking with a dog who is fearful and aggressive, we must have peace inside — not fear or anxiety over how the dog is going to act. This peace will get through to the dog; it will dissolve all fear.

Cindy came to understand that the jaguar drawings and objects in her home were not there by chance. We know the future, since we are unconsciously creating it all the time.

"The Sparrow's Gift" confirms that when you choose life, miracles happen. Talking about miracles — a sparrow pecking disease away — imagine that! The bird was debriding the wounds, removing unhealthy tissue from the woman who had shown the bird compassion. Animals have feelings and relationships that are meaningful to them. They feel your love, they know you care, and they go to help you with something. They communicate by their actions.

The gift — the rose — reminds me of a woman who

was undergoing chemotherapy, and when she left the hospital after her treatment, she'd vomit all the way home. Her husband would hand her the bag he kept in the car for that purpose. One day as she readied herself to vomit, she opened the bag and found a dozen roses from her husband. She told me she never vomited again during the rest of her treatment. What a beautiful gift of love.

In "The Divine Within," Klaus teaches the same thing I learned from Amelia Kinkade (see Amelia's story on page 186). Through pure communication the women and animal become united. It's not the physical union, but the recognition of their spiritual nature as one being. Humanness is not our only nature; people have to realize we have a *second* one — the divine nature. Don't be afraid to express your second nature. We are all capable of changing and finding that divine nature, using love as our weapon. It's not that we're changing who we are; we're just shifting into a higher spiritual gear and working at a different energy level. I call it the journey: it affects our beliefs, our environment, and all kinds of things. You can't stay the same from minute to minute. That's what the journey is about. When you're willing to shift, to change your nature, you move closer to the divine.

"Targeted by Dolphins" illustrates the higher level of connection and awareness in these great ocean creatures. As Jenny learned, the dolphins sense the problem and do what they can. Animals respond to their intuition; they don't let their intellect confuse the issue.

I knew a young woman named Michelle who had extensive cancer and went to Florida to die. She had some therapist friends who introduced dolphins to kids who had various injuries or genetic problems. The kids would go in the water, where they would be touched and loved by the dolphins. Michelle contacted me to say it was amazing. The dolphins zeroed in on the parts of her body where the cancer was. They left her with such a wonderful feeling, she didn't die. She came home again, feeling so much better. Two years later, far exceeding her expected survival time, she called me, saying, "I'm ready to die now. I'm tired and ready to die, but it isn't working. You say it's easy to die, but I'm having trouble. It's not happening."

I often say to people it's not hard to die. You can turn off the switch. When you want to live you keep it turned on; when you're ready to go you turn it off. At the end of our conversation I reminded her of the dolphins and how they don't think; they just do what feels right. Then I said to her, "Michelle, I've never had a phone call from a dolphin." That night I got a call from her parents to thank me. She had died quietly that evening. Reconnecting her with those dolphins had made all the difference in the world, empowering her.

We all send out sonar messages, often without realizing it, and these can be therapeutic or destructive. Studies have shown that patients who felt their doctor's compassion recovered faster than those whose doctors didn't answer their questions or communicate with them. Love is the most powerful sonar and can even be felt by strangers. Try it. Send love messages to a stranger you pass on the street. Many times the stranger will smile at you because they receive and feel the sonar message you are sending. Use humor as sonar too. When I park my car in an attended lot, I'll often say, "When I return I'd like to go home in a Cadillac." One guy responded, "Do you have a color preference?" We laughed and had a hug. Now the world is a better place.

How often, when we see someone is in trouble, do we go over and say, "Can I help you? Can I hold the door for you or carry your luggage?" We stand there and think, "Oh, that's terrible." I say: Go out there. Send out your sonar — I mean it. Be like the dolphins. Send your love and let it radiate around you. Many people will sense it and respond. Lives have been saved when people feel loved, because you show them you care. As one suicidal young lady said to me, "You're my CD, my Chosen Dad." She's alive and well today.

10

The Psychic Connection

I don't know what you should do with your life. But
you do. Your desires are God's desires trying to manifest
through you. Act on them.

— Amelia Kinkade

We can't explain how the universe was created.
Who or what created the existence of everything
in the cosmos? How did living beings evolve from basic
elements? Where did our consciousness come from? It
is there around us all the time. When our intellect gets
in the way, we can feel separated from our connection
with the source of creation. But if you quiet your mind
and have faith — which amounts to trusting that you
will know when you are ready — your awareness grows.
That's the nature of life.

In the Bible where it says, "In the beginning was the
word, and the word was with God, and the word was
God" (John 1:1), replace "the word" with "consciousness."

There is no question in my mind that consciousness is God, as are love, energy, and intelligence. All those are part of, and essential to, creation.

Since consciousness is within and around *all* of us, it is being picked up by others whether we are intentionally sending it or not. It is usually experienced as an instinctive or subconscious knowledge, such as animals knowing, when they first come into a home, how they will be treated, or patients going to a doctor and sensing whether the doctor has compassion and a connection with people.

A defining trait of consciousness is that it isn't confined to a specific locality, such as the physical brain. Quantum physicists and other scientists describe consciousness as "nonlocal," and this nonlocalness explains the ability of people and animals to receive communication from "God-knows-where." I've had mystics bring me messages from the dead — saying things they couldn't possibly know about my life and the people I've cared for. Yet the messages and information they relate contain details that can be confirmed, details from the past, present, and future. I have also had healers lay their hands on me, healing a painful injury that I had been experiencing for months.

When you read the following stories, you may find yourself asking, "How could that be?" You don't have to accept or believe anything written here. But if you're open to allowing that these authors *experienced* what they have written, you may be surprised. When we open a closed door, greater awareness comes in. Who is knocking at your door? I invite you to open it now.

On Death and Transformation

Janet Elizabeth Colli

Sugar, our beloved cat of fourteen years, died yesterday. It was a year of slow wasting. Always there seemed to be hope of recovery right around the corner, even until Sugar's final examination, two days before her death, when Sugar had ceased to eat.

When she first lost weight a blood test revealed hyperthyroid disease. We started her on the recommended medication and were duly warned that the hyperthyroid condition could mask kidney disease. Sure enough, Sugar did not regain her weight.

When she was in her prime, Sugar's plump body gave her gait an unmistakable waddle. Short and stocky, she was the genetic legacy of her mother, Shalimar, a beautiful, long-haired Himalayan. The tortoiseshell kitten lived with her mother in a tribe of semiwild cats routinely fed by our neighbor. After losing our tortoiseshell cat, Tinkerbell, Sugar seemed heaven-sent. About ten months old, she still closely followed her nurturing mother. She would not let us touch her, shyly keeping just beyond our reach, until we used that universally irresistible cat-catcher, string. Finally we caught her, placed her in a carrier, and brought her home to our apartment.

Sugar's transformation, upon entering the brave new world indoors, was complete. She loved us immediately. There is nothing like a tamed feral cat's unconditional love. She exhibited no shyness with my husband, Tom, and me. But she spent that first night with her head tucked into a dark corner by our bookshelf, oblivious to the fact that we could see her chubby behind poking out. How funny that she startled at ordinary objects. A belt on the floor was obviously a snake in disguise!

Twelve years later when Sugar's health started failing, I engaged the services of Leigh, a gifted woman who employs healing touch. Leigh's sessions began even before she left her house. Leigh explained that an etheric Sugar entered her awareness through the subtle realm on the morning of the session. Leigh believed that even when she was sensing our beloved cat at a distance, Sugar was aware of their bond, somehow linked by the sheer intention of healing. Indeed, Leigh's hands would get hot before Sugar entered the room. Sugar would come in, sashay around Leigh's chair, and be stroked by Leigh's hands at each turn. At a certain point in each session, Sugar clearly lost interest and would head toward the door.

"She's had enough," Leigh would sagely respond.

"Really?" we'd wonder. Or was Sugar simply bored?

Leigh's last session convinced me that her interpretation was sound. Sugar was losing ground; feeling desperate, I called Leigh in. Surely she could stop Sugar's descent. Unlike previous times, Sugar refused to come to Leigh's side. Tom picked her up and held her in his arms, in this way allowing Leigh to gently stroke her, doing what she could. But when given her freedom, Sugar headed toward the door. Before leaving the room she stopped, turned around, and looked lingeringly at Leigh.

"She's saying, 'Thank you, and good-bye,'" said Leigh.

I broke then, for my denial was shattered. Sugar was already preparing to leave her body, leave her family and her life. She was ready to go. We made the decision with her veterinarian, who agreed to come to our house.

The day before the vet came, I arrived home after work and immediately went to attend to Sugar. What happened next was subtle, but real. Since I practice meditation, I am accustomed to altered states of consciousness. Even so, this happened as suddenly as if I'd stepped off a ledge and dropped to deeper ground. My thinking mind turned off. I became aware of a deep silence within the room as I regarded Sugar, and I took my place next to her on the couch.

A vastness had entered the room, come to take Sugar home.

The next day we took Sugar outside one last time, following her as she rambled through "her" yard, content to sniff and sharpen her claws. It felt so right, seeing her in nature. Henry, a spirit guide who lives in the realm beyond our ordinary senses, was at Tom's side. He gave us instructions that would help Sugar's passing and assured us he'd be there.

With Sugar finally inside, our vet administered a sedative to calm her. Henry's presence was in the room, and I remembered his instructions to look into Sugar's eyes to stabilize her consciousness. Tom held Sugar in his arms. After the first injection Sugar quietly breathed, content in Tom's lap. That's when Henry told us, "Sugar is already an angel."

As the next mixture entered her veins, Sugar's heart slowed to a stop. The final release came suddenly, with a distinct sense of breathless liberation. *Tom actually felt Sugar leave her body.* He was astounded.

In answer to that age-old question "Where did she go?" Henry said he caught Sugar, held her, and "showed her the stars above." Henry assured us that Sugar was overjoyed to meet with her now-deceased mother, Shalimar, and other members of her feral tribe. Does "cat heaven" really exist? Tom can *sense* her there.

Henry says Sugar is now in a holding place, and if we meditate with a candle, the flame will help Sugar's soul find a suitable vessel and her way back home to us. So we light a candle and wait, thanking her for her love.

A Cat's Perspective

CINDY HURN

⤙⤚

My tabby cat, Isis, used to stick pretty close to me. We had a special bond, and she liked being involved in whatever I was doing. So much so that it was not unusual for her to follow me into the bathroom and sit patiently while I used the toilet. On one such day, there we were, sitting opposite each other. Catching her eye, I nonchalantly said, "Wouldn't it be interesting if you and I could switch places?"

To my utter surprise, in what seemed just an instant, I was suddenly in her body, looking out from *her* eyes, as she walked up to her litter tray. I saw that, unlike my clean toilet, her tray was dirty. I was shocked at what had just happened and a bit ashamed at the difference in how I kept our toilets, and it changed my attitude completely.

From that day on I always made sure to clean her tray after each use. There's nothing like a bit of embarrassment to make a clear point!

Captain Harris

Amelia Kinkade

~✷~

The gates slammed ominously behind me as the officer ushered me through the private entrance reserved for residents only. It was my second visit to Buckingham Palace. The autumn before, I had stood with the rest of the tourists, separated from the Queen's abode by imposing Guards and gilded iron gates.

Now, barely five months later, I was inside those gates, my floral scarf whipping in the crisp May breeze. London was a far cry from the hundred-degree-plus temperatures I weathered in my native Los Angeles, yet perspiration trickled down my chest. Tucking my scarf into my jacket, I hurried to keep up with the stride of the assistant Adjutant, Captain of these barracks. We crossed the palace yard, flanked on both sides by the Queen's Guard. Every ounce of my courage and talent was about to be tested.

As a corporate enabler and international translator, with a growing reputation for solving management problems and creating cooperative teamwork, I'd been brought in to troubleshoot on "official Royal business." The regimental Guard was having personnel problems. Some older employees were growing discontent, while a few of the new foreign recruits were having difficulties adjusting to their environment and workload. None of these employees spoke English.

Brass-buttoned sentries saluted and clicked the heels

of their shiny black boots as we passed. The assistant Adjutant ushered me inside the building and down a long corridor where the employees were stationed in cubicles.

"I'm not sure we picked the best time for you to talk to them," the Adjutant said. "We just served lunch."

"It's okay," I responded nervously. "Maybe they'll speak to me while they're eating."

"This is Captain Harris," the Adjutant said as we reached one cubicle. "His performance has been excellent for years, but lately he's been quite argumentative. He seems to have lost his spirit. He's not nearly old enough to consider retirement, but he seems discontented with his job. Ask him what the trouble is."

As I walked into the cubicle, Captain Harris was facing the other way, eating a bowl of oatmeal. When he saw me he did a double take and then turned back to his lunch.

"Oh, I thought you were a carrot," he said.

"What!?" I said, utterly bewildered. I'd worked with a number of mentally challenged employees in the past, but no one had ever mistaken me for a carrot.

"Your sweater," he said. "It's my favorite color." I looked down at the coral orange sweater under my beige cashmere jacket. The color formed the elongated triangle shape of a carrot.

"His peripheral vision is not very good," I jotted in my notebook, "especially on his right side."

"Did you bring me any carrots?" he asked.

"No. I'm sorry, I didn't. I understand you haven't been feeling yourself lately. Are you having problems with your diet?"

"It's boring," he said moving over to a plate of dry-looking salad.

"And your digestion?" I asked.

"Not very good since my coworker left. Have you seen the cat?"

"No, not yet. What color is it?"

"She's gray-and-white striped. She visits my cubicle at night. She's been cheering me since my friend got transferred."

"Do you know if there's a gray-and-white cat in this building?" I asked the assistant Adjutant.

"Oh, yes. That's Emma. I didn't know he liked her."

"Tell him everyone likes Emma," Captain Harris said. "She does wonders for morale."

"Ask him if he wants to retire," the assistant Adjutant urged me.

"Of course not!" Captain Harris answered indignantly. "I'm one of the Queen's favorites! I've won many awards! I could never retire. It would disappoint her. We have to practice marching in the parade this Saturday, and the entire team is counting on me to be in charge."

When I relayed the message, the assistant Adjutant's eyes bulged.

"Yes!" he confirmed. "They have a practice on Saturday. Well, if he enjoys his work, and he's looking forward to the big event, ask him why he hasn't been able to concentrate lately."

"Your boss has been concerned about your performance. Are you not happy working here anymore?" I prodded.

"I miss my friend, Bernard. He was in the cubicle on my left. We enjoyed working side by side and talking after work. The cocky little whippersnapper was so full of himself, he made me laugh and feel young again. I was just beginning to show him the ropes when they shipped him out. He got transferred to the beautiful countryside, while I got stuck down here. I want to go up there too. Or I want him to come back. I miss him terribly. We need to be together. Please tell him to bring Bernard back," Captain Harris said.

"He's lonely," I said to the Adjutant. "He gives me the name Bernard, who used to stand on his left. He says Bernard was shipped to the beautiful countryside, while the Captain has to stay down here all alone."

The Adjutant was speechless. When he found his voice, he responded, "Yes, it's true! There was a Bernard standing on his left! I never knew he meant that much to the Captain. Bernard transferred to Prince Charles's hunting facility in the southwest a couple of weeks ago. The Gloucestershire countryside is green and beautiful; all these boys have much more fun up there, hunting through pasture and woodlands. We ship them back and forth to give them a change of scenery. We thought the Captain was too old to enjoy such vigorous exercise anymore. That's astonishing! Whoever would dream he could call his friend *by name!?*"

What's wrong with Captain Harris? Why wouldn't he know his best friend's name? Is he senile? Is he deaf?

Captain Harris is one of the Royal procession Horses of Queen Elizabeth II. I was invited to Buckingham Palace in May 2002 to work with the Queen's Household Cavalry just as the Horses were training for Her Majesty's Royal Jubilee. A few days later, I was further honored by an invitation to Prince Charles's hunting facility, where I got to meet Bernard in person and give him a kiss on the nose. Animal lovers, have no fear. Both horses were joyfully reunited shortly after my visit. And I understand the Captain's positive attitude to his work returned in full measure.

Kali

CAROLYN MONACHELLI

≈⟨≈

Some years ago my son was living with me and working in New Haven, Connecticut, visiting brain-injured clients in association with his work in human services. On one street he visited regularly, a young cat, upon seeing his car, would always rush over to him and meow special greetings. He believed the cat was homeless.

"Mom, would it be okay if I brought her home?"

"Of course. If she'll come with you, bring her," I said, even though we already had two cats. I then quieted myself, mentally communicated with the cat, and said we would claim her, take care of her, and give her a name when she arrived at our house. *I knew nothing of the cat's description*.

In a moment I felt a connection and heard "Kali." I knew that Kali was one of the ancient goddesses, and my son and I both liked the name, so we settled on calling her that. I looked up the goddess Kali on the Internet to learn more about her and discovered she was a black goddess.

The next time my son saw the kitty, he picked her up and brought her home. To keep her calm, he turned on the car's tape player, not knowing what was on the recording. Immediately the song "We All Come from the Goddess" began to play. When my son brought her inside the house, I was startled to see *she was black*. That's when

I realized the cat had picked her own name and sent it to me telepathically.

We gave Kali a temporary home in a roomy cage in the basement so as not to disturb our kitties. They had their own territory and comfort zones, and bringing a third member into the clan would turn their lives upside down. Kali purred, rubbed, and made intense eye contact, conveying her thanks for being rescued. She always looked for affection first and food after. I told her about her new name and that she was related to the goddess.

We cared for Kali over the next couple of months, frequently taking her out of her cage for romps around the basement. She was cuddly and loving, and she knew we loved her. Every weekend I took her to an animal adoption event, where she was always the calmest of all the kitties. Eventually a kind lady saw her, fell in love, and adopted her.

Kali, our little black goddess, went to live in the country with the lady and share her comfortable home with her many cats. At last, she had her own family who loved her and treated her like the little goddess she was.

Bernie's Comments

Janet's cat, introduced in "On Death and Transformation," received the healing touch — the hot hands. While some people are uniquely gifted to do this, we can all conduct that energy.

When Furphy was young I used to take him jogging. After a mile or so I'd put him in the car, then run past the car a few times so he'd see that I was nearby. Then I'd take him out and jog again in short bits, so I wasn't exhausting him. These days, when he coughs owing to his heart problems, I lie down with him, put my hands on him, and picture him doing things he did twelve years ago, bringing that energy into his body so he can heal. He's sixteen or seventeen now. Imagine that.

The hard part is making the final decision, the guilt you feel when you don't communicate with them and you keep second-guessing your decision afterward. That guilt is lifted if we know they're ready to go and are grateful for help.

My own inner guide is named George. I first saw him during a meditation. He has been seen standing next to me when I lecture; several people have drawn his picture, confirming his presence. The other day I was out shopping, and I heard people saying, "Oh look, there's Dr. Siegel. Hi, Dr. Siegel!" I said, "Please, don't call out my name; if I do something crazy, everybody will know who

I am. I don't want to be identified." So this woman said, "Okay, I'll find another name — George — I'll call you George!"

No coincidence. I went back and told her about my guide.

"A Cat's Perspective" illustrates the nonlocal trait of consciousness. When our mind is quiet, we can know another's thinking. At night I stand at the door and send a thought message to our cat: "Hope, I'm worried about you making it through the night. There are predators, we live in the woods, and it's getting dark. Please come in." It's amazing, but after sending out the message I wait a minute and I hear her calling, "I'm here, let me in." If she doesn't like what I'm thinking, such as "I'm taking you to the vet for your checkup," she disappears. As long as I think loving thoughts, she shows up. So my message is: "I love you; I care about you." And she comes.

Why would Cindy even ask herself, out of the blue, "Wouldn't it be interesting if you and I could switch places?" Was that thought initiated by Cindy, or was she connecting with her cat's mind? Since Cindy was being quiet and her heart was open to her kitty, the latter is possible. When we receive thoughts from another source, we often assume they have come from our own mind.

"Captain Harris" is typical Amelia. I'm so impressed with her ability and the way she teaches, proving we're all capable of communicating with animals. People see for themselves and can't deny what Amelia's doing; they try the exercises, and as long as they are open to what she's teaching, they're changed by it. Amelia's psychic communication with animals wasn't something she grew up with, but was a skill she learned after attending a workshop led by an animal communicator. When we put in the time, effort, and energy, we achieve our potential.

It's like the time I was operating on a man and his heart stopped. The anesthesiologist said, "We can't resuscitate him." I just spoke out loud to the patient, saying, "Jimmy, it's not your time yet. Come on back," and his heart started beating again. Everybody in the room said, "We like working with you; we were ready to get the gurney and carry him away." But a medical student who was present said, "That can't happen." I wasn't going to argue with him, but it is what happened. It was just too different from what he knew for him to accept.

In "Kali," the cat recognized her own divine nature, knew that she came from the goddess, and chose her name. The song that played in the car, confirming her name, was no accident.

When our rabbit, Smudge, died, I drove to the vet to bring her home and bury her. I was grieving and also felt guilty about my part in her death. I had just decided that listening to music might help me, when I noticed that a new tape, given to me by a handicapped friend, was sitting there; so I popped it into the player. What's remarkable is that it didn't start on the first song, but halfway through the tape. The message of the song was that there is a universal plan for every woman and man, and that we second-guess ourselves, not understanding why things go so wrong, even though we try to do the right thing. There are reasons for our paths going the way they do, and there's no such thing as a mistake, only the lessons we need to learn. Those lyrics were like therapy to me.

Why was the tape sitting there? How did it come to play the middle song first? My message is that life is a journey we create, and any curse can become a blessing. The charcoal of life, when submitted to pressure, becomes a diamond. We are here to live and learn and raise the level of consciousness, creating a better future for all.

11

Talk to the Animals

Being a therapist for animals is no different from being a therapist for humans, except animals often respond and heal more quickly.

— Amelia Kinkade

Once you have experienced communication with an animal, it opens a door to a whole new way of being. Even if you can't hear what animals are saying to you, you *can* just talk to them. Tell your dog or cat what you want him to know. You don't have to speak the words; just say them in your mind. Before you leave the house, mentally tell your dog or cat how long you'll be gone and when you expect to be back. Picture yourself walking in the door and giving your animal a hug. Ask him to take care of the house while you are gone, so he feels he is helping you. If your animal likes music, turn on the radio and tune it to soft music. When you return, thank your friend for taking such good care of everything. You'll be surprised how much this helps your animal be less anxious about your being away. When you see that animals really do understand, you'll wish you had begun communicating with them sooner.

Years ago our kids came running into the house, saying, "There's a big snake out there, and we're afraid it's going to bite us." I quieted my mind, mentally went to the snake, and said, "Please assure me that you won't bite our children, so I can tell them and they won't be afraid to come out." The snake communicated to me in return: "Okay. Tell them I never intended to bite them." I went in and told the kids, "Don't worry; the snake promised not to bite you. You can go and play."

A week later I noticed the kids having a wonderful time in the yard, and I went out to thank the snake. I found him all bruised and entangled. I asked, "What happened to you?" He said, "Your kids. They knew I wasn't going to bite them, so they started playing with me, and look what they did to me." I apologized to the snake and said, "I told you I didn't want you to *bite* them; I didn't say you couldn't hiss at them."

Be clear about telling the animal what you *want* to have happen, not the reverse. If you tell your dog, "Don't run into the street," she might act upon your mental image of her running into the street. Instead, tell your dog, "Stay next to me and be safe when cars pass by." Picture her staying by your side. Talk to your departed animals too. Their consciousness hears you and will come to support and love you when you need them.

The following stories involve people who verbally communicate with their animals, and whose animals make it clear they understand. Read the stories, then go and tell your animals how beautiful they are and how much they mean to you. You might be surprised at their responses!

Heart Therapy

Leslie Green

One afternoon, my friend Anne brought her eleven-year-old dog, Pickles, to my practice. He lay limply by her side, like a rag doll with no stuffing. Ever since his sister, Peppers, died, Pickles had refused to eat. They'd been together since birth. Anne had resorted to feeding him with a syringe, but she couldn't get enough in to sustain him. He'd grown so weak she feared he too would die. Distraught, she tried using Emotionally Focused Therapy, a form of human therapy that involves tapping the body while recalling emotional trauma, and reciting affirmations that help the brain to resolve the trauma and heal emotional wounds.

"He still isn't eating," Anne said, sighing. I watched my friend tapping along her dog's spine and wondered if Core Health and Heart Forgiveness techniques would work with a dog. Most energy healing involves something done "to" the client, such as in Emotionally Focused Therapy, Reiki, and other types. But the Core Health technique teaches people how to release issues themselves and return to their core of pure health.

As an advanced facilitator of this technique, I use a method that includes forgiveness from the heart and energy level of every cell, which enables people to clear out stored anger and other baggage. This method is the most effective I've seen for assisting people in releasing these issues and mastering their own energy. I have counseled hundreds of patients at an alternative cancer treatment center, using this technique and utilizing the philosophies of Dr. Bernie Siegel, Dr. Bruce Lipton, Gregg Braden, Louise Hay, and others. For years I've been documenting successful outcomes, many in which patients became cancer-free.

When I asked Anne if I could try it on Pickles, she responded, "Yes!"

People need to forgive another for dying. Core Health recognizes that this process has several parts, beginning with the "will to live." Rarely does anyone's will to live measure 100 percent, yet in order for an individual to heal, it must. The next part of the process is called heart forgiveness. This forgiveness is easily done once all the issues are identified and released. But how do you discuss loss, anger, and grief with a dog? Knowing that energy connects us all, I sat in my chair and muscle-tested Pickles, substituting my body for his as he lay nearby on the couch. His will-to-live measurement was 20 percent. I tested him to pinpoint the time when he lost his will to live, and it turned out that it was one year previously. Anne confirmed this, saying, "That's when Peppers died."

I tested for a number of issues related to losing his will to live, and then, as I would with a human, I spoke to him out loud. The following is a much shortened version of our session.

Relax, close your eyes, feel yourself being in your heart and in every cell of your being.... See yourself standing in front of you, and connect your heart with that younger heart of yourself.

See all the baggage you picked up around choosing not to live. See it falling off your back, being pulverized into a fine, powdery mist; watch as a breeze comes along and blows it into the universe; let every cell feel it leave as your body returns to the healthy energy of the universe....

Now see each cell in your heart light up and radiate outward until every bodily cell is bright and joyful.... See this happening from your head down to your paws.... See Peppers standing in front of you, and join — heart to heart — with her.... Tell her you forgive her for dying.... Feel your two hearts joining as one.... Feel her energy and essence join yours....

Now see the road into the future. See yourself joyfully walking on that road with Anne and with Pepper's spirit.... Feel how free and light you are, expressing the true you.... When you are ready, open your eyes, bringing this with you, forever and ever.

Pickles lifted his head and looked directly at me for quite a while. The energy flowing between us was far greater than any energy I've ever felt flow from human to human. Gratitude, joy, and peace emanated from him. Then he looked at Anne, climbed into her lap, and snuggled in.

When Anne took Pickles home he ran straight to his food dish and began eating. He gained ten ounces in seven days and continued with a healthy appetite from then on. Pickles returned to his normal self! Anne was ecstatic. The next time I saw him, the vibrant Pickles ran over and danced circles around me. He'd never done this before.

This transspecies communication was the most profound I have ever experienced. The love flowing between Pickles and me was rewarding, humbling, and wonderful. It is clear to me that there is a strong connection between our species, and healing can be the result. He didn't have to understand what I was saying, for energy and connectedness exist in all sentient beings, including plants.

I love seeing people change from a state of anger to a state in which they allow life to flow. Being privileged to work with people at the most intimate and sacred times of their lives gives meaning to mine. And experiencing this healing of a dog that, while suffering grief and intense emotional pain, was starving himself is indescribable. If Pickles can be helped, so can others. Every positive shift in one being raises the energy of all beings. Overjoyed for Pickles and Anne, I'm also deeply grateful for this experience because it changed and shifted me too.

Asta Grass Joy

LISA L. OWENS

≈⚬≈

When Asta's racing career ended at age two, Tim and I gave the beautiful white-and-fawn greyhound a forever home. She gifted us with ten special years and unconditional forever love.

Behind the adoption kennel's grating, Asta had seemed little more than a shivering body, expectant hazel eyes, and a perpetually panting tongue. She'd been labeled "nervous," and no truer assessment has ever been made. As one of her longtime health-care providers liked to say, "Asta has her concerns," the simultaneously most endearing and exasperating of which included paragliders, toasters, and just about any noise that followed more than a minute's silence.

Asta was anxious during our meet-and-greet walk until she spotted lush grass growing through the kennel-yard fence. She snatched a mouthful, then spun around to show us her ill-gotten greens, so happy and proud! Some dogs eat grass only when they're feeling sick, but this young lady simply loved her salad. We knew she'd picked us the moment she tried to share her joy.

Later, we trained her not to touch neighborhood yards, but she'd often perform a fake snap just above the lawn, then look back and check to see if we got her "Asta grass" joke. We always did. Joyfully realizing we shared her sense of humor, Asta played this game on nearly every walk.

I like to say that Asta chose us…or that we chose her *because* she chose us. But the truth is there was no tangible decision. We simply knew we were a family, and that was that.

We said good-bye to our sweet girl early last fall. Tim once said that she and I were so close we shared a heartbeat. He wasn't far off. I could always read her body language, mood, and intentions, and she could read mine. Asta was my office assistant, my best buddy, my 24-7 companion, my baby. It was a privilege, during her final moments, to rest one hand on her head and the other on her precious heart, right up until it played its last beat.

Last spring we felt ready to open our hearts and home once again. Choosing a new dog was a daunting prospect. We couldn't expect another lightning-bolt bond such as the one we'd had with Asta. Worrying that the pressure to get it right might cause us to freeze during the selection process, we took a deliberate, systematic approach, narrowing the field of adoptees' Internet photos and biographies from around thirty to ten, then to three, and down to the final two.

I was drawn to Ewan well before meeting him in person. His burnt-umber eyes and beguiling expression in the photo stunned me. Something in this handsome face made me want to know what made him tick. During our selection visit at the kennel, we asked to meet Ewan first. I was deeply charmed when he leaned on me the second we met. His name stayed at the top of my personal list. But Tim and I had agreed beforehand to consider the other greyhound too, and so we met another wonderful boy, one who, we felt, based on his background, would have an easier transition into life as our pet. We knew we'd love him. He was a doll.

While I compared my final thoughts about Ewan and this other dog, my instincts kept poking at me, urging me to just go ahead and bundle Ewan into the car. Could I trust my gut?

That's when I silently asked Asta to send me a sign if Ewan was right for us and if we were right for him. At precisely that moment, the other canine contender gobbled up a little grass and looked off into the distance, not at us — no connection with us to share the joy. It was my sign!

Asta had given Ewan the nod, reminding me to trust that I know true love when I feel it. Just as she had playfully stolen that first bite of grass, Ewan had unreservedly rested the full weight of his body against mine.

As Tim and I shared our decision with the kennel staff, a leashed Ewan marched me straight over to the facility's front entrance. One volunteer laughed, saying greyhound residents used that door only when leaving with their new family.

"He knows," she said. "And he wants his car ride home."

Ewan got that ride. Now our home is filled with a big and busy brindle boy who, in many ways, is Asta's opposite. While she was light, he is dark; while she was shy, he is outgoing; while she was a finicky eater, he's game for sampling anything — footie socks and iPods included. Thanks to angel Asta, we finally have another forever love to call our own.

Telephone Rescue

SCOTT FRIED

⁓⚬⁓

Peppy's jet-black curls always bounced, a sign of our fifteen-pound miniature poodle's high energy and zest for life. He loved with enormous passion and played like there was no tomorrow. All the canines who had preceded him in our household had been German shepherds, and we raised him the same. We never thought to alert him to his lack of size and weight. Peppy was extremely intelligent, a loyal friend and fierce protector who did everything and went everywhere with us, even on our boat.

Later in life Peppy began to go blind. Dad taught him to pace off the rooms in the house, and Peppy navigated accordingly, running around as he always had, even after he'd gone totally blind.

I was fifteen when Dad, at forty-seven, suffered his first heart attack. While he was in the hospital, Peppy stopped eating. He lay around and refused to play or run. When several days passed and Peppy still hadn't eaten, we became almost as worried about him as we had been about Dad.

Seeing my father's improvement, we finally decided to tell him about Peppy on one of our visits to the hospital. Dad sent us home immediately and had us call him. He told us to put the phone to Peppy's ear, and Dad talked to the dog for about fifteen minutes. Peppy seemed to recognize Dad's voice and even what he was saying.

After Dad hung up, Peppy immediately ran over to his food bowl and began to eat. From then on he was fine.

I learned then that animals mourn just as strongly as we humans do. They feel the same emotions, they love, and they form connections just like us. I learned from my father that we can heal our animals, just as they heal us, with unconditional love. The relationship is a two-way street; but most humans attach conditions to their love. When we observe how our quadruped family members love us without reservation or provisional requirements, we learn better how to heal one another and how to live life in a more loving and peaceful way.

Love Talk

DORIE WALDEN

≈≈

Shabba was a pure-white cockatoo with a sulfur-yellow crest and paler yellow feathers lining the underside of his wings. As he grew, he developed a large vocabulary, which he used frequently. It included his name (his favorite word), our names, and those of our other pets. His language went beyond the repeating of words or phrases that we taught him. He would take words we had said or that he'd heard on TV and change them around, often into grammatically correct sentences that were appropriate to the moment.

Shabba also made up little songs, ones that always featured his own name. His singing was in the style of words spoken in rhythm rather than sung. He would also ask simple questions, such as "Hey, Dorie, where ya goin'?"

He would call each of our cats and dogs by name, praise them, scold them, and even mete out punishments. If one of the dogs did something that Shabba didn't think was right, he would send the poor animal into his crate — something we never did. Moreover, the dog would do whatever command Shabba ordered, and more quickly than he would ever do for us!

During the sixteen and a half years that we had Shabba, three of our other pets passed away. Once they did, he never called for them or spoke of them again.

Somehow he knew, when their last visit to the vet occurred, that they would not come home. He would be subdued for a period of time after their passing. When he did speak during this mourning time, it was primarily to express affection and give support to us.

Shabba could be incredibly perceptive about people. One day I was cleaning around his cage, which was in the living room. As I worked, Shabba asked, "Dorie, what's a matter?"

"Shabba, Dorie doesn't feel well today," I said.

There was a slight pause before Shabba said, "I'm sorry, Dorie. I love you."

"I love you too, Shabba," I answered.

Shabba then said, "Kiss, kiss, kiss."

I was so touched at his sensitivity and love that I had tears in my eyes as I went to his cage and gave him a real kiss.

Even with his limited vocabulary and meager grammatical training, Shabba was capable of expressing exactly the right thing at the right moment. Although we taught Shabba his vocabulary, he taught us so much more, not the least of which was about understanding and responding to others with love. Although he is no longer with us, I always think of him and say, "God bless you, Shabba," and I thank him for being such an important part of our lives.

Bernie's Comments

Leslie Green's story "Heart Therapy" reminds me of a book called *You Are the Placebo: Making Your Mind Matter*, by Joe Dispenza. Quantum physicists now recognize that desire and intention alter the physical world, causing things to occur that otherwise would not normally occur. It's incredible that when you create healing images, such as an image of every cell in your body lighting up, the body believes it is happening. Studies have shown time and again that even though it begins in the mind, physical change occurs. When people visualize themselves exercising, their bodies get measurably stronger and healthier, as though they had done the exercise.

In one study they put students in front of a machine that generated a repetitive movement. The students were told to slow the machine with their thoughts. Others were told to speed it up with their thoughts. A control group of students simply watched the machine. The researchers measured a significant speed difference in the machine's movements in the presence of those who visualized either more or less speed. Other studies involved healers sending loving energy to water. Results showed that plants fed with the "loved" water grew faster. Our intention and desire do make a measurable, noticeable difference.

Leslie treated Pickles like she treated human patients — no difference. When we speak words to an animal, our images and feelings connected with the words transfer through waves of consciousness. When animals get love from their owners, therapists, or other living beings, this helps restore them to their healthy state, because the animals' body chemistry changes.

"Asta Grass Joy" illustrates how a relationship with a loved animal or human endures, that their consciousness remains. People are often afraid to ask their dead loved ones questions. Lisa wasn't. She asked which dog was the right one, and Asta responded. We need to get over the fear of doing so-called crazy things; and when we are open to trying, surprising and wonderful responses can happen.

In "Telephone Rescue," Scott's dog weighed only fifteen pounds, yet he became their protector. We had an Irish terrier named James Cagney, and when I'd go jogging, he'd come too. Despite his small size, if a big dog was in somebody's front yard, he'd run up to it and bark. I knew James was doing that to make sure the dog didn't come after me as I went running by. That always impressed me, that he had no fear. It's the same with this little guy, Peppy: they had self-esteem, self-worth.

When I was out lecturing I used to call home. Bobbie would hold the phone up so everybody (meaning our animals) could hear me. They'd all relax. Animals instinctively know that the relationship works both ways: love benefits the giver and the receiver.

Dorie's story, "Love Talk," reminds me of our daughter. Carolyn still has cockatiels: they hear people talking and they learn. Carolyn and her husband would call out to each other in the house, and the birds would learn to mimic their voices. One day, Roy heard Carolyn yelling, "Roy!...Roy!" And he yelled back, "Why do you keep calling me? What do you want now?" Another time, Roy's voice yelled, "Carolyn!...Carolyn!" And she kept yelling back, "Yes, I'm here. What is it?" But they discovered it was one of the birds mimicking their voices. After that, Carolyn and Roy had to figure out if the voice they heard was that of their spouse or a bird. This gave new meaning to the statement "There's a third person in this marriage."

Our editor at New World Library, Georgia Hughes, used to play the bassoon in a woodwind quintet. Rehearsals took place in the home of the clarinetist, who had two birds. One of the birds used to whistle along, imitating the flute's part, even learning complicated pieces, like "Stars and Stripes." This bird also mastered the greeting on his owner's answering machine. If the phone rang when the man was home, he'd pick up the receiver, but before he could utter a word the bird would launch into the greeting: "You've reached Robert, and I can't take your call now. Please leave a message at the sound of the beep. (Pause) beeeep." The imitation was flawless, and despite Robert's attempt to convince callers he was home, they'd leave a message and hang up.

Dorie's story brought the words *one soul* to mind. When we feel that connected to each other, we heal each other. Scientific studies have shown that when you are surrounded by loved ones, you feel less pain. Try it yourself — put your hand in a bucket of ice and sit alone in the bathroom. Record how long you can stand to leave your hand in. Then do it again while surrounded by your loved ones. You'll be surprised how much longer you can leave your hand in the ice.

According to Jewish tradition, every visit by a loved one takes away a percentage of your disease. They can't cure you, but each person carries away some of the pain, a little of the discomfort or disease, and replaces it with love. That's what Dorie's bird was doing. You can actually feel your own body chemistry change when you think of the bird's comforting words, "Kiss, kiss, kiss."

12

Animals and Dreams

Your dreams, what you hope for and all that, it's not separate from your life. It grows right up out of it.
— Barbara Kingsolver

Peoplе have always been fascinated by dreams. What are dreams? Where do they come from? Are they merely chemical changes in the brain? Are they nature's way of helping us practice survival skills, and assimilate experiences gathered during the waking hours? What about dreams that seemingly predict the future? Can the spirits of people and animals talk to us in dreams?

In recent years, scientific studies have made use of neuroimaging equipment to study brain activity during REM sleep (the stage of rapid eye movement), a time when dreams are most commonly reported. In such studies, the images of brain activity recorded during REM sleep are compared to neuroimages taken when the subject is awake. During wakeful consciousness the visual cortex, located at the back of the brain, becomes highly active. When dreams happen during REM sleep, the visual cortex shows similar activity. Neuroimaging has also revealed that the same visual pathways activated during dreams and conscious wakefulness become similarly active when we visualize or imagine something in detail.

Consciousness is not restricted to the physical brain. Communication of intelligence and energy may *utilize* the brain, making it possible for our senses to see, hear, feel, and smell, just as a computer screen enables us to transmit, watch, and listen. The computer is not the source of the message; it is merely the mechanism that transmits the communication.

I have had dreams that made me understand that the fear of death isn't what led me to become a doctor; and when I had symptoms that could have been because of cancer, I was told in a dream, "but you don't have cancer." And I didn't.

The following stories may challenge your beliefs, and they will certainly touch your heart, for they show that when love exists, dreams do come true.

The Bridge Is Love

Audrey B. Carlson

Despite the happiness in our household, my husband always reminded us that he was outgendered and outvoted by the female majority. Bruce would jokingly raise both hands for the male constituency, against those of his two daughters, two female dogs, and me. We were blessed with much laughter and joy. Tragically, all this would change when our daughter Elizabeth was murdered. After she was taken from us our lives spiraled downward.

Desperate to find some way through the anguish of our loss, I embraced anything that might help. Shortly after Elizabeth's death, Bernie Siegel entered my life. He became my mentor, teaching me important mantras to live by. One came from Thornton Wilder's *Bridge of San Luis Rey*. Bernie pulled the tattered book out from his collection. Having seen better days, it was secured with a rubber band. He thumbed through worn pages and then pointed to a passage. The single line spoke volumes and resonated deep in my soul: "There is a land of the living and a land of the dead, and the bridge is love."

As I drove home, I remembered those words. I knew that keeping those whom you love in your heart and mind, and maintaining your unwavering, unquestionable belief in their presence, keeps love alive forever. As I repeated the phrase, I noticed the sky was unusually blue, almost crystal clear, except for the area directly above me where a long, connecting bridge had formed between two large clouds. Stunned, I pulled over and stopped the car. It was the bridge of love!

I soon became immersed in studying the spirit world. One day I asked Bruce to consider inviting Elizabeth into his dreams. Bruce, an engineer, saw things as black or white and struggled with the gray of the spirit world. I suggested that he merely invite Elizabeth into his dreams and trust the process. But his puzzled look made it clear he needed help.

"Okay," I said while looking at my husband. "Elizabeth, would you please come to Dad in a dream and — metaphorically speaking — hit him over the head with a frying pan and say to him, 'I am right here, Dad!'" Bruce smiled. I repeated that he didn't need to understand but should just trust the process.

Months later Elizabeth came to Bruce in a dream. Standing close to him on fresh green grass and holding a standard poodle puppy close to her heart, she said, "Daddy, here is the little boy dog you always wanted. When your life changes, he will come to you as a gift." Elizabeth put the black puppy down, and it scampered over to Bruce.

Bruce suddenly woke and couldn't go back to sleep. Waking me, he related the dream, which had been powerful and profound, and his emotions were palpable. I told him to remember her words, "When your life changes…"

Two years after Elizabeth's death, Bruce took early retirement. We decided to visit my mother in Florida, and so we boarded Giselle and Charlie Girl, our two standard poodles, with our breeder, Ann Fisher. Ann had been a breeder for over thirty years and had a full house of poodles.

After returning from Florida we went to Ann's to pick up Giselle and Charlie Girl. Inside her house, Ann gave one command, and all of her poodles came to attention — all except one. This black poodle ran straight over to Bruce, jumped into his lap, plopped two giant paws on his shoulders, put his nose against Bruce's nose, and began the most heart-wrenching sobs I've ever heard from a dog. Bruce, also feeling intense emotion, held the dog close, and a few seconds later Bruce began to cry. Then Ann cried. Something incredible was happening here — something that needed to be understood. Ann took a deep breath and began to explain the unexplainable.

Three weeks before Elizabeth was killed, she had come to Ann's to pick up Giselle from a grooming appointment. Ann mentioned there was a new litter of puppies, and Elizabeth asked to see them. She picked up all the puppies, one by one, saying she was looking for just the right male dog to buy for her dad. She found him, only to be told he was the pick of the litter and had already been spoken for. Disappointed, she returned home with Giselle. Elizabeth never told us about what she'd been planning to do.

Aries, the male puppy that Elizabeth had desired for her dad, came back to Ann two years later to be put up for rescue. He was the same dog that had come to Bruce in the dream and was now in his lap, crying to finally go home. He did come home with us that day and has not left Bruce's side since. He sleeps with us, reminding us not only that spirit can communicate through dreams but also that the power of love makes this possible. Love is eternal. Love *is* the bridge that connects us all.

The Vision Board

MARK S. KUHAR

My daughter always wanted a cat. Being allergic to cats and having always been a dog person, I always said no. But my daughter is remarkably persistent, so she kept asking for a cat, and I kept saying no.

One night we were creating vision boards, where you cut pictures from magazines that represent what you like and want in your life, with the hope that they will become manifest. My daughter put pictures of cats on her vision board.

"Good luck with that," I told her. "We are not getting a cat."

Days later my wife went out to take the dog for a walk in the park. She never brings her cell phone along, because she doesn't want to be disturbed on a peaceful walk. The odd thing is that on this particular night — the only time she'd ever changed her routine — she slipped the phone into her pocket before she left the house.

As she entered the park, my wife heard desperate meows coming from the top branches of a very tall tree. Following the sound, she spotted a little orange cat, alone and scared, looking down at her. It was calling to her for help. Remembering she'd brought the phone, my wife immediately called me.

"Come to the park and bring a ladder," she said. "There is a cat stuck in a tree."

Without thinking, I responded to the tone of emergency in my wife's voice, threw a ladder into the van, and drove straight to the park. By the time I got there, my wife was already holding the cat. Despite the presence of our dog, the little cat had climbed down from the tree, gone to my wife, a total stranger, and attached himself to her leg. He was not going anywhere.

"We have to keep this cat," she said as we got back to the house. Of course, my daughter was elated.

"We should try to find its owner," I said, and went out to drive around, looking for signs that someone might have posted for a lost cat. There were none.

In the meantime, my wife and daughter brought him into the house. Our dog sniffed him with anxious dismay, then walked away, as if the cat belonged there. They gave the cat some milk; he was obviously starved. Needless to say, we kept the cat.

Oddly enough, I have never felt any allergic symptoms since the cat came to live with us. Even more surprising, "Bigg" has become my best buddy. He constantly jumps onto my lap when I am working in my office, and he sits with me every night in my chair when I watch TV. Bigg is part of our family. It never ceases to amaze me that it all started with a picture on my daughter's vision board.

Boceifus

KRISTEN WEINDORF SHORT

My husband and I married and moved to Maine in 1988, and for the first time in nearly twenty years I didn't have a dog. It felt strange, but the demands of our hectic work and school schedules would have been unfair to a dog; it just wasn't the right time to adopt. The years passed with many moves, work changes, and the arrival of two of our three children.

In the spring of 2005, I dreamt that the four of us were hiking in the woods on our property, and a male yellow Lab walked beside me. I looked down and our eyes met. His gaze was so kind and wise; it seemed that my heart already knew this loving creature. Upon waking, I harbored a deep sense that a special dog was coming into our lives. When the circumstance presented itself, I would know it was meant to be.

Weeks later a woman whose children attended my day care told me about her sister's yellow Labrador retriever, named Boceifus. Her sister loved the dog dearly, but a broken relationship and, subsequently, her demanding work schedule meant the year-old pup was often left alone. Although hesitant to give him up, she felt it would be best to seek another home for him. Tears welled up as I recalled the dream of the yellow Lab with the expressive eyes. My special circumstance had arrived.

Boceifus swiftly became a much-celebrated family member, accompanying us almost everywhere we went. Loving and loyal, Bo's one great anxiety was being left alone. Since I worked from home and the kids were there, he was rarely alone.

Bo and I shared a special bond from the beginning. He followed me everywhere. He lay by my feet when I was working and slept near me at night. On occasions when I was away from the house, he'd wait by the door until I returned, even though the rest of the family was home. He would look at me with those expressive eyes, and I always knew what he needed. Somehow he always knew what I needed too.

In 2007, Bo welcomed our third child into the family with wagging tail and wet kisses. Then, on July 15, 2010, the joyful atmosphere of our home took a cataclysmic blow. My husband, a family practice doctor, delivered news that no doctor wants to give to any patient, let alone his wife, and which certainly no one wants to receive: "You have cancer."

This silent breast cancer had evaded screening and diagnostic imaging, enabling it to grow over many months. A biopsy revealed the ugly truth. I crumpled into my husband's arms while Bo nuzzled my tear-moistened hand. My journey had begun.

After the cancer diagnosis, Bo remained close to me, both in physical proximity and in spirit. In my darkest hours he lay at my feet or snuggled against my body. He patiently endured long days when I was too weak and tired from treatment to do anything, and he expressed his joyous gratitude when I felt well enough to take walks and throw the ball for him.

In 2012, we decided to adopt a yellow Lab puppy, which my daughter aptly named Nutmeg. Bo lovingly tolerated the young pup's playfulness; he even joined in at times. But his personal mission of watching over me remained his top priority.

In the ensuing eighteen months, Bo became increasingly frail as he developed stiffening joints and had difficulty catching his breath. He still wanted to sleep near me but had trouble mounting the stairs. He'd sit at the bottom step and look at me with those expressive eyes. Now I was helping him up the stairs and settling him in comfortably for the night in loving gratitude for all his years of kind companionship.

In June 2014, we drove to Pennsylvania to visit family. The kids, my husband, and I gave Bo and Nutmeg special hugs as we left them at our veterinarian's boarding facility. The long car trip in tight quarters would have been hard for Bo, and we sensed that having Nutmeg there would help him during his stay.

Three days into our trip I received a harrowing phone call from the veterinarian, telling us that Bo had suffered a critical health crisis. He was alive but sedated, and his prognosis was guarded at best. Deep in my heart came the overwhelming knowing that he was waiting for me, just as he always had.

After a seven-hundred-mile, prayer-infused drive

back to Maine, we arrived at the animal hospital. The veterinary assistant looked at me with tears in her eyes. "He's waiting for you."

"I know," I whispered.

It was bittersweet and beautiful to hug my beloved friend, whispering words of love and gratitude in his ear. "I'm here, Bo."

When our eyes met for that last time, he sighed, and I felt a great, gentle wave of peace flow through him. We all showered him with our love and tokens of affection. I remained with him, holding him, thanking him, as they gave him his final injection. Bo passed peacefully in my arms. That night and for many days after Bo's passing, Nutmeg was visibly subdued.

The void he left behind was huge. Oh, how I missed my dear friend. One morning I woke to a compelling sense that Bo was with me. Had I dreamed of him again? I glanced down to the foot of the bed, and there were kind, wise eyes gazing back at me, only these eyes were young. Nutmeg was lying by my feet, filling the void Bo had left behind. Bo remains a source of guidance for her. Somehow she always knows when I am sad or feeling unwell. Seeking me out, she snuggles up; and those beautiful, expressive eyes are still watching over me.

The Dream Diary

SANDY WEINBERG

❧

Max came with my husband as part of a package deal when we got married. Having spent his first years as a bachelor's outdoor dog, Max reveled in his new good fortune. He enjoyed lounging on the couch like a prince in his palace. He didn't want to be outside unless we were with him. Although initially my husband's dog, Max soon adopted me. He became unashamedly a momma's boy. He was my shadow, my companion, my buddy and protector.

Max was a force of nature, crazy with energy; many of his characteristics came straight from the pages of *Marley and Me*. No amount of walking tired him out. My husband had been assured that his yellow Labrador would outgrow puppy behavior by the time he reached the age of four. Then it was: "He'll calm down when he is five years old," then six, then seven, and so on.

The word *incorrigible* was invented just for Max. Nothing was safe when he was around. We couldn't leave the house unless it was "Max-proofed" first. If I was cooking, Max was patiently waiting for his moment. As soon as I turned my back or left the kitchen for just a second, he was counter surfing or table thieving, absconding with whatever delicious morsel he'd been eyeing. Max was helpful too. When I loaded the dishwasher, he happily provided the "preclean" cycle. Never tiring, he'd come in after a long walk, and before long, I'd be chasing him around the house, pulling some item out of his mouth. He just couldn't help himself. There were so many trips to the emergency veterinary hospital that we learned by heart the instructions for how to induce vomiting in a dog.

Max never slowed down until he reached eleven, his last year, when he became ill. It was heart-wrenching to see this once hearty dog struggle just to walk up the stairs. Almost overnight he went downhill. When he was diagnosed with pulmonic stenosis, we took him to a cardiologist, who put him on medication that caused him to suffer hair loss. Patches of skin showed clearly through his sparse yellow fur. We tried homeopathic remedies, and I gave him Reiki and Reconnective Healing treatments; but in the end his body was failing, and it became clear that it was time to let him go. After Hurricane Sandy we had no electricity, and I was nursing my dying dog all week with no power, a cruel twist of fate. On November 4, 2012, we lost our beloved Max.

It was torture coming into an empty house the first days after Max was gone. The house felt so lonely without him. Every corner contained a void that Max and his boundless energy used to fill. I didn't want to rush into getting another dog, so I learned to get used to the quiet.

People told me that Max would send us our next dog…that he would choose. We thought we'd wait at least six months before seeking another dog. But when February heralded the approaching spring, I started to get the bug. I searched online rescue groups and found Labs4rescue and our new dog.

We welcomed Bentley into our home on March 10, 2013. He was a one-year-old black Lab, originally adopted by another family, who were giving him up. If it was Max who sent Bentley our way, he must have known we needed a break, because he sent us a dog that doesn't grab things off the table, surf the counter, or steal from the kitchen sink. The house no longer feels lonely. It is alive with the love and energy of a new pup.

I have kept a dream diary for several years, and about a month after adopting Bentley I suddenly thought of a dream I'd had several months before. I ran upstairs to get my diary, and I found this entry from December 24, 2012:

> Dreamed of Max: He's lying on his side, fur sparse like it had been, but whatever we've done in the dream (stop medication or start one?) it results in some hair stubble starting to grow back. The stubble is black, and I'm wondering if he is now going to be black instead of yellow.

This meant that seven weeks after Max's death — more than two months before we started looking for a new dog — the wheels that would bring the black-furred Bentley to us were already in motion. That dream had come to me on Christmas Eve. Was Bentley our gift from Max? If he did have his paw in this, I wouldn't be the least bit surprised.

Bernie's Comments

In "The Bridge Is Love," when I read that the dog Elizabeth had picked out came running to her dad and jumped into his lap, I burst into tears. We all need to be loved; love is the only thing of permanence. When sharing that quote from Wilder's book, I used to recite more of the paragraph, beginning with: "We ourselves shall be loved for a while and forgotten, but the love will have been enough." Our love makes us immortal. The daughter's thoughts and feelings were communicated and were felt by the animal, so he ran to the dad and jumped into his lap. It's no accident. Audrey helped Bruce to heal with her suggestion about asking their daughter to come into his dream. And when she pointed out Elizabeth's words, "when your life changes," it gave her husband hope. Hope opened the door.

"The Vision Board" shows that love is the best medicine, even for allergies. The cat delivers a dose every time he sits on Mark's lap. When Mark says, "I'm not allergic anymore," it's because he's become different. He accepts the cat, so his body doesn't respond with an allergic reaction. He changed his body chemistry. When the mind creates an emotional reaction or negative belief about something, it produces messenger molecules that activate genes. A substance called histamine is released, inducing an allergic reaction. But when you change your attitude, the brain produces different chemicals, so the reaction is different.

The daughter's vision board helped the girl to imprint on her subconscious the image of what she wanted in her life, and that blueprint of consciousness created the future she desired. Images make up the language of the unconscious.

In "Boceifus," Kristen had a dream: the Lab walked next to her and looked into her eyes, her soul. She connected to the dog through the dream. Dream images are like drawings, often revealing the future. Subconsciously we know the future. It's all mapped out, and time — as we know it — doesn't exist. Animals teach us: "Don't worry about the future; go for a walk, have a treat, whatever it is that makes you happy. We're still here — let's do it!" When Kristen was okay, Bo reflected that energy; when she wasn't, he supported her. Bo's spirit trained the younger dog. When Nutmeg took Bo's place on the bed, Kristen knew she was not trespassing but filling the void. Nutmeg was able to live in the present, instead of focusing on what was missing from the past, and that became a source of comfort and healing for Kristen.

In "The Dream Diary," when Max changes from gold to black in her dream, Sandy becomes ready at a subconscious level to recognize the black dog and accept him into her life.

Her story about Max helping to wash the dinner plates reminded me of a time our grandson came to stay with us. I was putting food on the table, and he said, "These plates aren't very clean."

"That's as clean as cold water can get them," I said. Later he stepped outside and saw a great big dog we had recently adopted, one he hadn't seen before.

"Grampa, there's a big dog in the yard."

"Don't worry, he's friendly," I said. Then I stood in the doorway and yelled, "Hey, Coldwater, come in here!" Bobbie loves Coldwater; you put anything on the floor — pots, pans, plates — and he gives them the prewash cycle.

Keeping a dream diary helps bring subconscious knowledge into the present. One night I dreamed of a sparkling, iridescent cat. Its name was Diamond, but nobody in the dream pronounced the *d* at the end. I couldn't understand why they weren't saying it right. My therapist friend, James Hillman, later told me the cat's name was Daimon, and he represented my spirit and soul. Finally I understood; I got the message. It was very powerful. The dream diary becomes a guide, another tool for understanding, changing, and healing your life. By keeping the diary, you let your unconscious know that you are ready for its messages of wisdom.

13

Grief and Forgiveness

In grief we can be more connected to loss than grace. In grace we restore the relationship through forgiveness.

— Elisabeth Kübler-Ross

During World War II a German bomber dropped its load on Bristol, England, then turned south and headed back toward Germany. Hit by antiaircraft tracers, the plane crashed in a valley in Exmoor, killing all but one of the men. The surviving aviator, a lad of seventeen, crawled out of the wreckage and climbed to the top of the hill. Alone in enemy territory, he had no idea where he was, could not speak English, and expected to be killed or taken prisoner. When a farmer walked into the field, the young airman put his hands up in surrender. The farmer stopped, noted the German uniform and the boy's frightened face.

"I 'aven't time for fighting," the farmer said. "I've got

me ewes to tend to." He strode past the young man, disappeared down the field, and left the lad wondering, "Now what do I do?" The dazed airman kept walking until he found somebody willing to take him prisoner.

These people eventually adopted him into their family, and when the war was over the German boy married a local girl. The people created life, not war, out of forgiveness and love for another human being. Animals understand this without thinking about it. They teach us that we are the same at both ends of the rifle.

One evening when I went to bring the animals inside for the night, our rabbit, Smudge, was snuggled up to Furphy, the very same dog who had attacked and wounded her the previous year. Smudge had not only forgiven Furphy, but was now best friends with her attacker. Imagine that. When Smudge died from a complication caused by her old wounds, I couldn't forgive myself for having left her alone with Furphy only days after their introduction. By forgiving Furphy, Smudge was also showing me that I needed to forgive myself. We aren't perfect; we don't know everything; we miss things we should notice; and we make mistakes.

Sometimes in our grief over losing one animal, we withdraw from loving another. Our fear of hurting again results in their going hungry for love. But as with Smudge, the animals forgive us.

The following stories show how forgiveness isn't about forgetting, but is about accepting that whatever happened was in the *past* and moving on — not fearing the future, but caring for those who need our love now.

Saving Grace

Veronica Leigh

∽≈

"What do you think of these?" Mom asked. My sister and I bent forward to get a better look at the computer screen displaying three basset puppies available for adoption.

I shrugged. "They're okay."

Two months earlier Casey, my golden retriever, had died of cancer. The last thing I wanted was another dog. Sensing I was less than enthusiastic, Mom dropped the matter.

In November she brought up the subject again. This time she had a two-year-old basset in mind. The dog was at an animal rescue shelter in Kentucky and desperately needed a family. Again, I wasn't interested.

"Pray about it and let me know," Mom said.

Casey hadn't been gone a year and already Mom was looking for a replacement! That really hurt. At the same time, Mom seemed to have her heart set on this dog. Was it right of me to hold back just because I couldn't let go of Casey? Casey never held back from anyone when it came to opening her heart. "Okay, get the dog," I told her.

My family drove down to Kentucky and came back with a scrawny, awkward-looking creature. Her belly sagged and swayed from having multiple litters, and she left slobbery-gobbers on our pant legs and furniture. Her name, Sunshine, didn't suit her, and she refused to come to it. I remembered a basset hound named Grace in a children's book series, so we tried calling, "Here, Grace!" and she came. She liked it.

Days after her arrival, Grace's collar broke while she was out walking with my sister, and she ran off. My sister chased after her, but it was no use. Grace was gone. We thought we'd never see her again. That night, our cat alerted us to a noise on the front porch, and when Mom opened the door, there was Grace sprawled out on the glider, waiting for us to let her in.

Grace fit in well with the family. I slowly grew to love her and forgive her for not being Casey. Mom hadn't been thinking only of me when she suggested that Grace join our family. She had hopes for Dad as well. Dad always liked the family animals, but ever since the death of his English sheepdog, a loss that had broken his heart, he'd remained somewhat aloof toward animals. Dad's mother had recently died too, and now rumors about layoffs at Dad's place of work added worry to his grief.

There was something special about Grace that began to work a miracle inside him. Her presence made the hard times a bit easier to bear. We'd tease him about loving her, and Dad would respond by saying, "She's all right, for a dog."

She must have been more than all right. This was the dog he shared his food with, took on walks, called "the baby," sang songs to, and even allowed to sleep on his bed.

The years slipped by, and the aging Grace, with stiff joints and white hairs framing her muzzle, seemed right with the world, until Dad suddenly passed away. His absence confused her; she moped around the house as we all tried to cope with our grief. In spite of her loss, Grace tried her best to comfort me. In the two years since then, she and I have grown especially close.

I thank God for bringing Grace into our lives. I don't know what I would have done without her. She never took offense at my reticence to accept her, but she showered me with love until I learned to love again. I've come to realize that I needed Grace as much as she needed me.

Second Chance

KAY PFALTZ

When my first dog, Lauren, died, all I wanted was to follow her. I thought the pain of grief would never leave. But sometimes in life we are given a second chance to live and love. My opportunity came when my friend Patty called to tell me, "Kay, there's a sick beagle at the SPCA. She's scheduled for euthanasia."

In Virginia beagles fill the shelters, many discarded when they're no longer able to hunt. But I didn't want another beagle after Lauren. I wasn't ready. And I had Flash, a tiny smooth-haired dachshund with a huge personality and even larger spirit. I wanted, at least for a while, to lavish him with the attention reserved for an only dog.

But something behind Patty's pleading was saying, "You can make a difference…at least in one life."

When I arrived at the shelter, I was taken to the isolation unit. A volunteer opened the door to a motionless heap on a blanket. This looked like no beagle I'd ever seen; covered in hairless pink sores, she had a seriously neglected case of mange. Unlike the rich tricolor of my beloved Lauren, this small creature looked like a dingy gray dish towel that someone had wrung out and dropped. I knelt down. The eyes in that poor little face glanced at me once and then quickly away.

"She's sick…and deeply depressed," the girl said with a shrug that implied, "We can't save them all."

A vision flashed before me of this abandoned dog euthanized for no fault of her own, her final days in a cement run, knowing no love, only discomfort and pain. Didn't she deserve a chance? The fear of opening my heart again only to have it battered once more made me decide not to adopt but to foster her after she was no longer contagious with mange.

Hardly a week after Chance came home as a foster dog, I realized how attached I was growing to this small dog with the domed head and Chihuahua eyes. Emerging from her shell of despondence, she would shadow me. But on the day she followed me into the bedroom, I shoved her away, not wanting to love again, not wanting to hurt.

Flash and Chance were soon inseparable. She grew independent and strong, a second mother to Flash, a gentle teacher to me. She didn't need to follow me around anymore. She knew me inside and out. We communicated easily without words, me intuitively sensing her thoughts and desires, and she knowing where I was and when I was coming home.

As the months passed, I realized this dog wasn't the only one to receive a second chance. I had often been overprotective with Lauren for fear something would happen to her. Finally I was learning that it had never been up to me to decide Lauren's fate, and it wasn't for me to decide that of Chance or Flash either. I could love them and offer the best care possible, but I had to let them live and do what they loved doing. Flash wasn't as prone to follow his nose when hunting and run off, so it was left to Chance to break my fear.

The years took their toll on Chance. There was the panting and coughing at night, and I learned patience. There were trips to emergency vets in the cold morning hours, and I learned to trust. There was the double snakebite requiring intensive care for nine long days and nights, three blood transfusions, and a plasma transfusion to save her life. The experience ultimately forged an even deeper bond between us. It was Chance who comforted me when Flash lay on our bed and took his last breath. And Chance was there to welcome into our lives Sasha and, later, Olive — two more dogs in need.

The day that I shoved Chance away was over twelve years ago. So independent then, Chance once again follows me from room to room, like in those early days. Her deafness forces her to search with nose and waning sight for the comfort and reassurance of knowing I'm here. Words can't express the love my fingers know every time they caress the lumps and bumps that cover her fragile frame, or the feeling that wells within as I stand and watch her sleep. I love her more than I have words to say. The only thing I shove away now is the ache I feel when confusion shadows her white face.

Every time she tries to jump up on a chair and falls, or she walks the wrong way while searching for me and stares into an empty room with pricked ears, she breaks my heart — just as I always knew she would, again and again — each break making more room for the love.

Loving animals opens me to my best and most tender self; now I always let in love. Thank you, Chance, for a second chance at getting life right.

Joy Coach

KATHY SDAO

❧

The first thing you should know about Effie is that her fur is so soft it will startle you. You'll be compelled to rub your palms slowly along her sides and press your cheek against her velvet ear. You'll catch a whiff of her scent, an intoxicating mix of moist earth, turkey meatloaf, and fleece beds; and you'll run the risk of having your face pummeled by her big slick tongue.

DNA testing asserts Effie is part Brittany spaniel and part Labrador retriever, a Blab — or if you prefer, a Litany. With her chestnut patches on white, she'd easily blend in with any pack of foxhounds hunting the moors.

The next thing you should know about Effie is that she saved my life. When husband number two announced monogamy wasn't really his thing after all, in a way so similar to that of husband number one, fifteen years earlier, that it seemed they compared notes, I plummeted into despair. This surprise revelation occurred on September 10, 2001. The next morning my anguish was magnified a hundredfold as the twin towers fell. In the space of twelve hours, previously unimaginable events had devastated my sanguine reliance on a stable marriage and a secure country.

I was a wreck. I bundled the shards of my shattered heart in a bubble wrap composed of friends, family, and faith. I could not accept that my husband, now living with another woman, was really leaving me. One winter night at 2 AM, I lay sleepless in Tacoma yet again, my relentless humiliation and looming loneliness eclipsing any sense of light. Hopeless, and so exhausted that breathing seemed too much work, I decided to pool all the prescription pills I could find in my house.

As I shuffled around, Effie followed. She watched. She stood with me in the bathroom wondering why we weren't in bed. As I sat on the edge of the tub, grasping once more for my seemingly absent God, Effie gently placed her bowling ball of a head on my lap. She kept it there as my tears soaked her muzzle. I grew aware, with genuine surprise, of a tiny ribbon of relief growing deep inside. The simple pleasure of her presence at a time when nothing else brought comfort was the first stepping-stone on my path back to wholeness and happiness.

Effie has been my joy coach ever since that moment. Her all-consuming bliss, when discovering for the several-thousandth time her beloved plush hedgehog on the kitchen floor, is a lesson in the art of living. She knows what's important: Play daily. Experience the nowness of every moment. Speak volumes without words, and surround yourself with dear friends.

Effie and I walk a few miles every morning. I treasure this time, when I can most easily pray. The beauty of my neighborhood combined with the absence of any sort of electronic screen frees my monkey mind to suspend its near-ceaseless chattering. During these walks, I've become aware of a different sort of prayer — simply enjoying the intimate presence of our extravagantly loving Creator. No words; no thinking; just being — being enough; being loved as is, despite all my mistakes and messes. Walks with Effie aren't just time to pray; they are prayer itself. My pure delight in this magnificent dog is soul work. It wedges open heart space that would otherwise seal tight and solidify into cynicism.

I adopted Effie as a pup from the Kitsap Humane Society on the first business day of the year 2000, meaning she is now fifteen years old. Our remaining time together is precious. Each morning that I awake to find her beside me and eager for another day's adventures, I shout, "Thanks, God!" for the gift of this living work of art, this indomitable angel — both blessing and balm. I love her beyond measure. I may not know how to pick men, but I sure as hell know how to pick a dog.

Fingal

ROWENA WILLIAMSON

Fingal came to me as a puppy with enormous feet and a tail that dragged on the floor. Although I'd had Scottish deerhounds for many years, Fingal was the first puppy. His name, based on that of the legendary Irish giant, had been decided before I got him. It was a perfect choice. I watched him grow tall as an Irish wolfhound; he could reach the middle of my chopping block without any effort and help himself to whatever food was on it. Fingal grew up, but he never grew out of puppyhood.

I already had Taz, a deerhound bitch, but when Fingal joined the pack, we bonded in a special way that was far stronger than I'd ever experienced with the other dogs. Fingal always rose early to join me while Taz still slept. I'd sit on one corner of the couch reading the morning paper, and Fingal, yawning widely, would perch on the adjacent loveseat, all four feet on the floor. He assigned himself to be my constant companion. Although he had flaws that kept him from ever winning ribbons — a massive overbite and a high ridge on his skull — he had a personality that drew people to him. Fingal was different. None of my other deerhounds had ever had his capacity for unbounded joy, his goofiness, and his need to be near me, something that made me grateful for every day with him.

When he was two years old Fingal was diagnosed with Addison's disease. For the next two years Karen, a wonderful vet, helped him through attacks that took his temperature to dangerous heights. There were also night-time drives to the emergency veterinary hospital when his life was threatened by a crisis. Fingal was loved by all the people who worked to save him. Stoic and with tail wagging, he put up with cold baths, injections, and being away from me and his mate, Taz, and he took his treatment with mute acceptance.

One morning Fingal wasn't quite his usual happy self, so I took him to Karen, who found an enlarged anal gland. She took care of it, and we said how nice that for once there was only something simple going on. That evening Fingal seemed restless, his heart's pounding visibly evident. I worried, watched him, and finally, when he settled down, I went to sleep. At five in the morning I woke up and found him dead. I learned later that the disease can produce high levels of potassium, which leads to a heart attack.

What followed was a period I find difficult to think about. We always feel guilt, I suppose, when a dearly loved pet dies, but my ties with Fingal were so strong, and we had gone through so much, that even now, as I write this several months later, I am once again in tears.

Fingal was a puppy at heart, though he was nearly four when he died. He would still come and bury his head in my side for comfort, and he'd try to climb on my lap when he weighed 116 pounds. Taz and I still mourn him. She lies on her bed and whimpers, and his big gray shadow seems to follow me, as he always used to do. When I think of Fingal and his goofy ways, I know our short time together was merely the introduction, for love never dies. One day we'll be together again.

Curmudgeon

CHELSEA WOLF

Robert opened the cage door, and the saddest little face I have ever seen immediately began to nuzzle my outstretched hand. This cat, rescued from the city pound just hours before being destroyed, was beginning his sixth month of residency at Robert's no-kill shelter in the East Village. The whole time I held him, he stared into my eyes. It wasn't until I put him back that he made a raucous meow.

"That's how he got his name," said Robert. "He talks like an old curmudgeon."

The fifteen months I had with Curmudgeon were like any serious relationship; it had its ups and downs. A trip to the vet revealed he was twelve or thirteen, and he came with a variety of health problems. They started off small — urinary tract infections and colds — and then became too big to ignore. There was blood in his feces; he vomited after every meal and eventually stopped eating altogether. Certain that these were side effects of stress, I brought him to a new vet, expecting to be sent home with antibiotics. Instead I learned he had an abdominal mass; these were the symptoms of intestinal cancer. I had been watching Curmudgeon die for months.

The last weeks were bittersweet. We sat and watched crime dramas together on the couch. Sometimes I looked into those sad eyes, and I knew exactly what he was feeling.

But other times I was at a complete loss as to how to help him. The vet said he wasn't in pain, so I planned on keeping him comfortable through the last days of his life.

Despite my preparing for Curmudgeon's decline, watching him die was one of the hardest things I've ever done. He hid under my bed much of the time. He lost a ton of weight and, with it, hair. When he did eat something, he threw it all up. He stopped using the litter box. One night I came home and found his pillow soaked in blood. I still don't know where that blood came from. I pulled Curmudgeon up on the bed with me and told him that if it was his time to go, then he shouldn't hold on for my sake. I also said if he needed any help on his journey to let me know, and we'd get through it together. He gave me head-butt kisses in response, and I knew he understood.

On August 21, 2012, Curmudgeon lost the ability to walk. At the twenty-four-hour clinic, the doctors rushed him into emergency care. His breathing was labored and he wouldn't stop crying. In addition to the mass in his gut, he had a blood clot that had broken loose and become stuck in the lower half of his body, paralyzing his back legs. There was nothing the vet could do to make him well, but he offered to try and stabilize him if that's what I wanted. I did not. I signed the paperwork giving permission to put my little fur baby to sleep.

I was with Curmudgeon in his final moments. He was sedated, wearing a catheter, and wrapped in a blue sheet. I told him he was a good boy, and I loved him very much. Then he nestled into my arm, the doctor injected him, his eyes got really big, and he was gone.

People say I have a love of broken things. Through-out my life I have tried, with varying degrees of success, to fix every one of these things.

I've often wondered why Curmudgeon came into my life, but I finally understand. I needed to learn how to live without being in control of everyone and everything around me. I needed to learn how to let things be and to keep moving on, even when it hurts — to love un-conditionally and uncontrollably, knowing full well that time with this loved one could end any day. Thanks to Curmudgeon I'm no longer afraid of loving or embrac-ing the brokenness in myself. I miss him so much, but I know that he's watching over me, filling heaven with his raucous old meows.

Bernie's Comments

In "Saving Grace," I like the name that Veronica chose for her dog, because of the song "Amazing Grace": "I once was lost but now I'm found…"

The dog and the dad make an amazing couple, helping each other to survive. When men don't have work anymore they often wonder, "What's the point of living?" But having a dog in the house gives them a relationship; petting the dog's fur releases oxytocin, the dog makes them laugh, and so on. The animal gives them another reason to live and a good feeling. I love the sentence where Veronica explains that Grace "began to work a miracle inside him."

In "Second Chance," I'm reminded of charcoal, which, under pressure, becomes a diamond, a beautiful gift. Any difficulty can be a blessing — a wake-up call.

One woman wrote on my website, "It's the anniversary of my husband's death, what should I do?" I said, "Go and do something nice for someone else. Don't sit there suffering; celebrate your love with deeds that bring lightness into the world. You can make a difference at least in one life." I found a small round badge the other day, the button kind that you can pin on your shirt. The message said, "One person can only do so much." A black line crossed out the word *only*. We can all make a difference. Kay did this when she agreed to foster Chance.

Years ago I had pins made up that said, "You Make

a Difference." When I traveled, if somebody did me a favor — offered their seat or gave good service — I gave them a pin. Their eyes would light up; and when they wore it, everyone who saw them got the same message. Take a chance; make a difference for somebody. Life requires your taking a chance when you get out of bed. It all depends on how you get up. If you make choices that support life, you're more likely to have second chances at getting life right. Kay chose to act selflessly, so it changed her and, now, the lives of everyone she meets. If we all did this, the world would be a miraculous place.

In "Joy Coach," I love the names Blab and Litany. Effie is like the God presence, the first step to wholeness. When animals are teaching you, you're seeing the truth — the wisdom. They are telling you, "Live today; you are lovable." When you feel loved, you don't consider ending your life. The animals do that over and over because they're not judging us. They love us *as we are*, and they see us as complete and whole.

In the story "Fingal," Rowena feels grief, loss, and guilt over Fingal's death. That's the sad part, when you feel there was something more you could have done but didn't know. We can all relate to her feelings; we all feel it. As for the time spent grieving, it takes time. But what if you're stuck there, holding on to it? Does Fingal think, "You must have loved me because you've been miserable for so long?" No, he wants you to have a nice day.

When my father died, I decided to wear black for the rest of my life, to remind myself of my mortality and the importance of living life every day. But after a while I realized, "This is really sick. Continually reminding your-self that you're going to die isn't healthy." Then I dreamed of my father; he was looking wonderful, healthy, and he was smiling. I woke up with a totally different outlook because he wanted me to smile, to be happy and enjoy the day. Now I wear colors that cheer people up.

Many years ago our seven-year-old son Keith had a pain in his leg. He requested an x-ray, which revealed a bone tumor. Shocked, I realized that the odds of it being malignant were high, and he'd probably lose his leg and die within a year. The next morning he came up to me and said, "Dad, can I talk to you for a minute? You're han-dling this poorly. I need you to help me have a nice day today and not worry about next year."

That's what animals are teaching us all the time. We can create an environment that leads to a life we can love while we continue to love our body, rather than feel angry at it for having a disease. Then our body gets the message. We were fortunate: it turned out that Keith's tumor was a rare, benign type.

In the next story, "Curmudgeon," Chelsea says, "I needed to learn…" The only thing you can control is what's going on inside your head. Animals understand this intuitively; that's why they don't need long lives like we do. We need to be comfortable looking at ourselves in the mirror and saying, "I love you," seeing not only the things that are wrong but also the miracle of who we are and all the things that are *right*.

As a physician, I felt guilty when I couldn't do any-thing to help my patient. I felt the pain and began to ask, "Why did God make a world like this?" But I had to learn that you can't cure everything. What you *can* do is care for everyone and help them to live *this day*. It's also good to let them know, "It's okay to die. You haven't lost the battle. You've lived; you've loved. You'll be immortal. When you get tired of your body, it's okay to leave. The love will stay with us. Learn to let go and let God."

As a surgeon, I was trained to handle disease, not feelings and loss. But we all need to learn how to turn the curse into a blessing, just as hunger makes you seek nourishment. It's about finding what's broken in your life.

It helps to ask, "Why did this happen now?" What is going on in your life? What factors are causing you a problem? Look at the cause. It's not about shame, blame, and guilt. When we learn something from our journey through hell, it isn't such a tough journey anymore because it's teaching us. It's a totally different feeling. I know this at a personal level. When I ask, "What have I learned from this experience?" I shift into a different place, and it feels so much better. I call that suffering labor pains — feeling broken is okay if it gives birth to something.

What lessons would we learn if the world were perfect? How would we grow if not for misfortune? It is only through an imperfect world that we find meaning in life. A perfect world would be meaningless, like a magic trick.

14

Life Goes On

A little while, and my longing shall gather dust and foam for another body. A little while, a moment of rest upon the wind, and another woman shall bear me.

— Kahlil Gibran

Following his son's death, my grieving friend took a walk in the Connecticut woods. A beautiful butterfly, unlike any he'd ever seen, followed him. It made him think of his son, who had loved, studied, and collected butterflies. The father took a good look at the insect, making note of all the distinguishing features. After returning to the house, he went to his son's room to look up the butterfly. It turned out to be a species found only in South America, yet the man had just been accompanied by one in Connecticut. He realized then that his son was saying, "I'm still here, Dad. I'm with you."

Once I was lecturing in Baltimore to hundreds of people, and I mentioned William Saroyan's stories, which capture simple lives and contain great wisdom and depth. That day, I happened to quote from "The Daring Young Man on the Flying Trapeze," where a young man finds a hotel room to die in. "The earth circled away, and knowing that he did so, he turned his lost face to the empty sky and became dreamless, unalive, perfect." That line always moved me with its stunning simplicity. After the lecture a woman came up to me and, with tears in her eyes, said, "I'm Saroyan's daughter. Thank you." It turned out this line had great personal significance for her. No coincidence. Her dad was saying, "I'm here."

The following stories illustrate life transcending death, and love with no beginning, no end. They teach that a part of us is in everything, and a part of everything is in us.

Three-Act Comedy

ANN CHESSMAN

~⚮~

Our youngest son, Paul, died at age nineteen in an accidental drowning. He was a quirky, funny young man, a ray of sunshine now gone, and I just couldn't deal with the loss. I spent an inordinate amount of time at the cemetery. There my grief had room to be whatever it was that day. Perhaps that's why I wrestled with resentment at dog walkers. They too had discovered this oasis of peace and beauty, yet they had the ability to go about living, while I was trapped in my grief.

All around me were signs of so much loss, but still I came. Paul would have been upset to see me sitting there, disconnected from the living world. But I couldn't help it. This was the last thing that connected me to him. I would tidy, replace, and water the flowers; I'd wash the stone of remembrance and enjoy signs that friends had visited.

One day I arrived at the cemetery filled with an extraordinary sadness. As I approached Paul's memorial, I stopped dead in my tracks, not believing my eyes. A flamboyant rooster and demure hen were circling around each other in the strangest courtship exhibition. Not only that, they were performing their act right on top of Paul's grave!

A day later I arrived to find a big cat sitting in the same spot, contentedly slapping the ground with its curled tail. How odd! The final act happened another day while I was refreshing the flowers. Suddenly a Steller's jay appeared and started bouncing on Paul's grave! It was a jubilant hoppy dance with head-nodding and tail flicking that lasted for a good three minutes. What was going on? Why were all these happy creatures invading my grieving space? The ridiculous antics of the jaybird suddenly struck me as terribly funny. Overcome by mirth, I laughed with abandon.

Two chickens, a cat, and a Steller's jay walk into a cemetery.... It sounds like a joke Paul would tell. Since none of the other graves boasted animal entertainers, it dawned on me that my son, or God, or the two of them together, were trying to say they didn't want me to lose my joy or spend too much time among the stones.

Those animals were indeed comforting to this mother's heart. They bridged the gap between worlds. Interestingly I've never been an animal person, yet I now have a tacit affection for the cat I adopted for my husband. It seems I stopped grieving and started living. Whatever would Paul say? I think my quirky, funny son would just wink at me and laugh.

Long John Silver

MARTHA POUND MILLER

In the forest Bonnie had stumbled across John's body — her husband, a victim of a sudden heart attack. Days, weeks, and months had passed in a blur. All she could remember of them was the pair of liquid brown eyes that had watched her constantly. It had been John's insistence on adopting the puppy — the one who licked the stump of its hind foot — that had saved the defective golden Lab from destruction by the breeder. They hadn't even named the dog yet when John died.

Bonnie woke to find that the trees outside her window had leafed out, and in the sunniest corner by John's shed, yellow daffodils seemed ablaze with color. She lay on the edge of the bed and yawned; the half-grown pup thumped his tail hopefully on the floor. Bonnie slid down, wrapped her arms around the shaggy coat, and breathed in his scent of wood smoke and dust.

"I haven't named you yet, have I?" she said. "Come on, let's go outside and check the garden." A tour of the yard revealed that some daffodils already needed deadheading.

"I almost missed spring," she mused. John would never experience another spring, and the realization hit hard. She crumpled. The dog's damp nose nuzzled her arm. She pulled him toward her and felt the sun's warmth on his fur.

"Nova," she said. At the sound of her voice, he stood at attention.

"Nova — sit." The dog dropped to his haunches, leaned forward, and licked her arm. Then he jumped up and raced in lopsided circles around the yard. His antics caught Bonnie unawares, and she laughed, surprised how her joy spilled over the grief. Looking at the newly named pup, Bonnie said, "You know what? John wanted to plant roses. Come on, Nova, let's go get some."

Nova sat next to Bonnie and watched the countryside whiz by. Old tree trunks, coated in velvet, glowed above fields of lacy ferns. The creek had cut a new path over the winter, running closer to the highway. As she passed John's favorite fishing spot, the ache of grief returned. Nova moved his warm body closer to her and stayed there until she pulled into Arthur's Nursery.

Mr. Arthur looked up from his potting table. "How's the mister?"

Bonnie's words stuck in her throat; she couldn't respond. When she got out of the car, Nova yelped.

"If I leash the dog, may I let him out?"

"Sure 'nuff," Mr. Arthur answered. "No good for a dog in the car on a day like this."

Her bad moment had come and gone. Taking a deep breath, Bonnie said, "My husband passed away last fall."

"I'm right sorry. He was a good man," Mr. Arthur said. After a moment's pause he added, "Nothing like new plants to keep you busy."

Bonnie found the roses she wanted and followed Mr. Arthur to the cash register, Nova limping along behind.

Nova halted at one of the display tables and nosed a scraggly rosebush in a can underneath. Bonnie tugged the leash, but Nova balked, sniffed the plant again, and sat on his haunches looking up at her.

"What's the problem?" she asked.

Mr. Arthur smiled. "He wants you to get that one."

"Looks like a reject," Bonnie said. "Nova relates to that."

Mr. Arthur lifted the sorry-looking specimen and set the can on the table.

"Long John Silver," he said, reading the label.

"What?" Bonnie's ears rang.

"It's a climber rose, but I meant to toss this one out. It just didn't grow."

"I'll take it."

"Heck, I'll give him to you. Let me know how he does."

Later Bonnie placed the Long John Silver can next to one of the patio posts. As she approached John's shed, her steps slowed. She opened the door and reached for the shovel. The wooden handle felt smooth and cool in her hands. She lifted the turf, and as she dug, the smell of black, loamy earth was so familiar her breath quickened. There was a rhythm to digging that felt good, and soon she'd made a big hole. She looked around for Nova, who was digging his own hole in a corner of the yard. She smiled. Something inside her seemed lighter.

After she had planted all the roses, her muscles ached and hands smarted where she'd pricked them. She showered and scrubbed her nails with a brush, then toweled off and put on clean clothes. Her stomach growled. She realized with a stab of surprise that she was actually hungry. Bonnie made a tuna fish sandwich and gave Nova his supper. He lay at her feet, black nose caked with garden dirt. John would have loved this runty little dog who had been slated for the vet's needle.

The first sign that Long John Silver would survive was the appearance of several young leaves. A few days later, a new cane emerged — fat and shiny — thrusting its tip toward the sun. By the next morning, it had grown an inch. Each time she looked, the vigorous cane had grown bigger. Bonnie decided to call Mr. Arthur.

"It's amazing," she reported. "The rose is growing like mad."

"He's happy there," replied the nurseryman. "He feels at home."

In a month, the climber was six feet tall and had two main stems with a multitude of branches lush with leaves. Bonnie had no explanation for why the rose grew so fast. Occasionally Nova lifted his leg on the other new roses, but he always spared Long John Silver. When the weather warmed, a profusion of small buds appeared, and soon clusters of white roses covered the bush, their fragrance filling the air.

One late-summer evening Bonnie sat under the bower created by Long John Silver. The sun dipped behind the trees and the light turned gold and mellow. Nova stretched out at her feet with eyes closed and heaved a great sigh of contentment. At the same moment a spent white rose released its petals in a soft cascade onto Bonnie's lap, and some landed gently on the dog's head. Nova's tail gave a single thump, as if responding to the touch of a loving hand.

"Yes, John," Bonnie said quietly. "It is time to start living again."

Saving One Life

Terry Persun

≈⊱≈

It all began when Cathy and I were living in Ohio and we attended past-life-regression sessions facilitated by a wonderful woman. In one session, Cathy revisited a life in which she, in an angry temper, had galloped off on a horse. During the ride the horse had spooked; she was thrown and suffered a terrible neck injury. That lifetime found her in a wheelchair, unable to care for herself. This explained a lot about my wife's current issues. Cathy has always suffered with neck problems and required monthly appointments with a chiropractor. All her life she had felt nervous around horses.

We didn't consider the connection between Cathy's problem and her past life until we found ourselves living on the Olympic Peninsula with a daughter who loved horses. Cathy often drove Nicole to her riding lessons at a local farm and gradually began to help brush and feed the horses and scoop manure. She even tried riding once or twice, but it wasn't an enjoyable experience for her. When Nicole started competing in horse shows, Cathy and I were around horses even more. While Cathy now felt more comfortable with them, her nervousness was still apparent. It wasn't until Annie showed up at the farm that things drastically changed.

The farmer's daughter went to see a horse that was for sale — the result of a nasty divorce. She found "Annie" in poor health, malnourished, and with a sore body from being stalled for long periods of time without exercise. Unable to leave Annie in that situation, she made a bid for the horse and brought her back to the farm.

From the moment Cathy set eyes on Annie she felt a kinship. Whenever she drove Nicole to her riding lesson, Cathy would spend time caring for Annie. Annie was in poor condition. Her fur felt crusty. Her hooves were in terrible shape. She was dangerous to be around if you made a sudden movement, and she threw her head and reared whenever anyone came close to her head. For all practical purposes, the horse was useless.

Cathy confided to me that she felt Annie was the horse from her past life, and she was determined to bring her back to health. It would be a big job. She wasn't even our horse. But Cathy's sincere interest was reason enough for me to back her in any way that I could. We made an arrangement with the farmer to take over the full responsibility for Annie's upkeep, though she would remain stabled and pastured at the farm. Cathy spent almost every day with Annie, and they got used to each other. When Annie's health returned, Cathy even rode her for a while. But then Annie's hooves began to have trouble, and the lame horse could no longer support a rider.

More than one person suggested putting Annie down, but Cathy refused. After doing a lot of research, Cathy decided to leave her unshod. She read about the work and recommendations of the best-known barefoot farriers in the country and even studied briefly with one of the natural hoof-trimming greats, Pete Ramey.

Annie's lameness was finally resolved, but her increasing age and the past difficulties she'd endured kindled Cathy's decision to give her a well-deserved retirement. One can tell by the way an older horse walks and moves around the pasture if it has any pain or movement limitation. Inspired by Annie's needs, Cathy studied and became a certified practitioner of Equine Natural Movement, taught by Joseph Freeman. She also mastered the techniques known as Hoof Rehabilitation and Equine Structural Integration.

Cathy continues to work with many horses outside the six that we now own. Her experience, knowledge, and ongoing studies keep her on the cutting edge of equine rehabilitation science and therapy, enabling her to help the animals she has learned to love so much. Amazingly, it all started with saving the life of one horse that Cathy felt a remarkable connection to.

We are deeply grateful to Annie for everything she brought into our lives and all she continues to bring. Because of a bond that crosses all understanding, one horse was saved from destruction, and many lives have been completely transformed.

The Unbreakable Bond

JANET PFEIFFER

The dog was huddled in the far corner of the animal shelter cage. I bent down and gently called to her. She approached, licked my finger, and wrapped her paw around my arm, tugging as hard as she could. A gut-wrenching cry, unlike anything I'd heard before, was her unmistakable, desperate plea to save her. I knew that instant she was mine.

Driving home with a forty-pound shepherd-sheltie mix perched in my lap wasn't easy. Her arms were wrapped tightly around my neck, and her chest was pressed against mine. Yet somehow, we made it home safely.

Halle had never seen daylight. Her footpads were as pink as a newborn puppy's, and her first walk on rough pavement caused them to bleed. Falling leaves and loud noises terrified her. Her coat was dull and brittle, her skin marked with hot spots, raw and bleeding. Seven years of horrific living conditions had compromised her immune system. Chronic eye problems required daily medication and soothing eye baths. Her front teeth, gnawed to the gumline on steel cage bars, were tiny brown stubbles.

Halle was a victim of medical research. For her entire life, she had been isolated in a barren cage in a laboratory. Like millions of animals around the world, she was subjected to unspeakable experiments conducted under the guise of science, and she suffered mental, emotional, and physical damage. Her only human contacts were the technicians who conducted the tests on her.

Halle was not fond of other dogs, but our other two rescues — Reba, a four-year-old shepherd-sheltie, and Buddy, a sixteen-year-old shepherd-Doberman — soon won her over. Reba's maternal instinct was to lick Halle's bad eye, a meticulous daily routine that gave temporary respite from the irritation. And Halle savored every minute!

Two years later, after the passing of Buddy, we welcomed a gentle shepherd mix named Sage. Having a new dog in the house, even one so enamored of her, caused Halle to become ill, to lose most of her hair and endure severe digestive problems. That's when I promised her that as long as she was alive, I would never adopt another dog, never subject her to any additional anxiety. Halle's well-being was my priority. Each night as we crawled into bed, I'd hold her close, tell her how much I loved her, and, placing a soft kiss upon her forehead, ask her never to leave me. I could not envision life without my special little treasure.

Periodically, I'd visit online rescue shelters. Halle was fifteen when I found an adorable black-and-tan puppy on Eleventh Hour Rescue's site. I fell in love immediately but knew in my heart it was out of the question. In spite of that, each night I would return to the site to see if the little black dog was still available.

Then without warning, our beloved Halle collapsed. I rushed her to the emergency vet, where they fought to save her life. Four hours later they gave me devastating

news: an undiagnosed mass in her abdomen had rup-
tured. Surgery offered a minimal chance of success and,
at her age, would be unfairly traumatic. I brought Halle
home in a box and buried her in our backyard.

Beside myself with grief, I spent the next two days in
bed, barely able to function. My baby was gone. I deeply
grieve each of my dogs when they pass, but the earlier
experiences had been nothing compared to this. There
would never be another like Halle, my once-in-a-lifetime
dog.

I forced myself back to work, but even in my pain I
could not get the image of the little black-and-tan dog
out of my mind. Five days after Halle's passing, I drove
to the foster mom's house. She brought the dog into the
yard and I instantly felt drawn to her.

"She's promised to another family," the woman said,
"but my instinct says she's meant to be with you." After
making a phone call to the rescue organization, she announced that the little girl was mine to take home. I was
ecstatic!

Willow immediately fit in with Reba and Sage. Within
days my husband and I noticed something strange. Not
only did Willow have markings similar to those of Halle,
but Willow also displayed more of Halle's quirky behaviors each day, odd mannerisms I've never seen in any
other dog. Halle, for example, could twist her body into
a pretzel shape when she slept. Willow slept in that exact
same position. Halle held her own leash when we took
our morning walk. Willow did the same. Halle used to
love snow. She'd bury her face in it, hold the position,

then emerge with a huge smile on her snow-dusted face. Willow too digs a hole, buries her face, and holds it for about fifteen to twenty seconds. Then, one day when I called Halle's name, Willow responded!

Could it be possible that Halle had honored my request never to leave me? I brushed it off as wishful thinking, until the day I noticed Reba licking Willow's eye, exactly as she had always done with Halle and *only* Halle. Willow had no eye problems.

Two months later, our Sage passed away. We adopted three more small dogs that year, and even though Reba loved all the dogs, the only one afforded the same care as Halle was Willow. Even Reba knew! I truly believe that, knowing we wouldn't adopt another dog while she was still alive, Halle selflessly "made room" for Willow, enabling the youngster to receive the same love and care we'd given to her. Miraculously, Halle's spirit found a way to inhabit the new dog, proving that our love bond was so strong, not even death could separate us.

The Reincarnation of Anka

CARMEN VAN ETTEN

I grew up in Germany in the 1960s. My parents always told amazing tales of Anka, a black German shepherd they had adored. But Anka died a year before I was born. Eventually I had my own dogs, and then one day I married and moved to the States.

My husband and I shared our lives with three wonderful rescued dogs. Late in the evening of February 2001, I was walking them in a park when I spotted a shadow in the woods. A thin black dog, wet and dragging her hind leg, ran away as I approached her. It took me four days, many treats, and lots of patience to finally catch her. At the moment she calmed enough to let me touch her, her eyes rested on mine, and I experienced an intense sensation of recognition. I was looking into the eyes of Anka, the dog whose stories had permeated my childhood. She limped to my car, jumped in, and spent the next ten years with me. I named her Annie. It was uncanny how she communicated with me without ever making a sound. After extensive surgery, she regained use of her hind leg.

My mother came from Germany to visit us a few weeks after I'd found Annie. When Mother walked into the house and saw Annie, she put her hands to her face, and shook her head, saying, "It can't be. It can't be — it's Anka!"

This dog was a Doberman–golden retriever mix. She

looked nothing like a German shepherd, but her gentle nature and expressive eyes revealed she was an old soul. Annie greeted my mother like a long-lost friend.

I never experienced anything like this before or since. We've had several dogs over the years and loved each and every one of them, but our relationship with the other dogs was nothing like that with Annie.

A powerful bond existed between her and me right from the beginning, one that remains to this day, even though she's been dead for almost three years. Annie (or Anka) showed me that love crosses all boundaries, including past, present, and future. I have no doubt we will be reunited somewhere, somehow, for it seems that even before I was born we were together, and long after she died we were reunited. Somehow our love endured time and conquered space; we were never truly separated.

Bernie's Comments

In "Three-Act Comedy," Ann's son presents a gift, something comical that would give her a different feeling so that she would start looking to life, not death and loss.

I built a stone cairn over the grave of one of our dogs and brought a rock to the site every morning as I walked by his grave. Then one morning I heard him say to me, "Why don't you bring me a flower?" So I picked a flower to place there. From that morning on I looked for beauty and stopped seeking cold stones. His words changed my focus and my feelings.

Because animals accept what is, they become natural channels for our loved ones who have passed. One woman in our cancer support group told us about her daughter who loved birds and who'd been murdered. When the girl's sister had an outdoor wedding, a bird landed in a nearby tree and made such a racket that people couldn't hear, and it interrupted the wedding. Everybody's reaction was "Your daughter is here." While she was telling this story to the support group, a bird flew in the open window. We'd been using that room for five years, and no bird had even bumped into that window, let alone flown in. Once again, people reacted by saying, "Your daughter's here."

In "Long John Silver," the husband's consciousness knew he was leaving and made sure his wife got the puppy before then. Our future is a part of our inner knowledge and wisdom. When you finally leave your body, there is no time: you're in the eternity of now. Your consciousness is ever present, so it can continue to communicate with loved ones for their entire lives, until you come together again, free of your bodies. Bonnie's husband communicated through the flowers. He was saying, "It's okay. Life goes on. I'm still here, growing a bower of petals over you and Nova."

When a star absorbs more matter than it can sustain, it explodes, ejecting its content in a burst of light, *creating new life.* This is called a nova. When Bonnie named the dog, the wisdom of her consciousness was saying that it's all about new life. A miracle of healing took place in this story, on either side of life and death; and in this instance, the dog became the connection.

"Saving One Life" brings up the age-old question of reincarnation. We are each impregnated with the consciousness of those who have lived before us. That a child is a prodigy at four years of age doesn't necessarily mean this child played the piano in a past life; she may have the *consciousness within her* of someone who was a pianist. If the consciousness within you may be part of what's causing you trouble, it's worth doing a regression through past lives. Life is a school. What is important is what you learn from the experience — do you spend your life avoiding horses? Or do you become a horse healer and bring something positive to the world as a result of your experience?

In "The Unbreakable Bond," Halle, the dog who died, impregnated the consciousness of Willow, the living animal. One of the women in our cancer support group had a son who had recently died. When he was alive, he loved pigeons. She told us that one night she was driving on the parkway when she heard her son's voice saying, "Mom, slow down." A pigeon landed on the lane in front of her car, forcing her to slow down to avoid it. As she came around the curve, twenty cars were piled up because of a sheet of ice. If she hadn't slowed down, she would have been one of the victims. Her son's consciousness had temporarily entered the pigeon, directing it to land in a busy highway, something pigeons wouldn't normally do.

Transplanted organs contain the consciousness of the donor. Recipients have often become aware of the presence within them that holds memories of the donor's life, and they recognize that this is a different person inside them. But it's easier for consciousness to enter the clean slate of a newborn or the nonjudgmental, open mind of an animal. My hope is that the consciousness we create in our lifetimes will manifest educating, life-enhancing thoughts and behaviors in those who follow us. If we learn from the difficult events in our lives, gaining wisdom and compassion, the next generation will become wiser and healthier.

The final lines in "The Reincarnation of Anka" contain a truth that animals teach us over and over again. "Annie (or Anka) showed me that love crosses all boundaries, including past, present, and future....Somehow our love endured time and conquered space; we were never truly separated." In a Saroyan novel there is a line that says, "Love is immortal and makes all things immortal. But hate dies every minute."

Threaded through the animal stories is the theme that where there is love, there is life, and love is immortal. The true miracle, the one the animals are always teaching us about, is love.

So listen to the animals. Don't wait for a disaster to happen before you decide to live your life. Animals are living the message of life, showing it to us even after they die. Pay attention to them. Go out, get a pet, and attend their school. Let them reveal what you need to learn. Let them expand your heart, and open your mind to the miracles that are waiting for you.

Epilogue

A sick man turned to me as he was preparing to leave the examination room, and he said, "Doctor, I am afraid to die. Tell me what lies on the other side."

Very quietly I said, "I don't know."

"You don't know? You're a spiritual man, and you don't know what's on the other side?"

I was holding the door handle, and just then we heard scratching, whining noises behind the door. As I opened it, Furphy sprang into the room and leaped on me with an eager show of gladness. Turning to the patient, I said, "Did you notice my dog? He's never been in this room before. He didn't know what was inside, except that his master was here, and when the door opened he sprang in without fear. I know little of what is on the other side of death, but I do know one thing: I know my Master is there, and that is enough."

Furphy died in his sleep shortly after that event.

Last Words

One more breath
How do I use it?
One more breath
Why bother? What do I tell them?
One more breath
Will they understand?
One more breath
What wisdom can I share?
One more breath
How can I enlighten them?
One more breath
I have the answer
One more breath of life
a-h-h-h-h-h-h-h-h-h-h
One more breath

— Bernie Siegel

Notes

INTRODUCTION

Page 1, *"Until he extends the circle"*: Albert Schweitzer, *Kultur und Ethik, Kulturphilosophie*, vol. 2 (Munich: Beck, 1923).

ONE: THE SIEGEL ZOO

Page 5, *"She filled her own mouth"*: Sterling North, *Rascal* (New York: Puffin Books, 2004), p. 26.

Page 16, *"What Is So Important I Can't Sleep"*: Bernie Siegel, "What Is So Important I Can't Sleep" (unpublished poem).

TWO: BECOMING FAMILY

Page 19, *"He needed the companionship of a family member"*: Ralph Helfer, *MODOC: The True Story of the Greatest Elephant That Ever Lived* (New York: HarperCollins, 1997), p. 252.

Page 19, *"of all nations, and kindreds, and people, and tongues"*: All biblical citations in this book are from the King James Version.

Page 19, *"Home is a place where"*: Robert Frost, "The Death of the Hired Man," in *North of Boston* (New York: Henry Holt, 1915), p. 29.

Page 20, *"guard the life of another creature"*: Lloyd Biggle Jr.,

The Light That Never Was (reprint; Rockville, MD: Wildside Press, 1999), p. 132.

Page 21, *"Awaken, My Love"*: Bernie Siegel, "Awaken, My Love" (unpublished poem).

FOUR: REVERENCE FOR LIFE

Page 63, *"A work of art"*: Bernie Siegel, "Red Squirrel" (unpublished poem).

Page 65, *"And if there's no Heaven"*: Edmund Vance Cooke, "Rags," in *The Best Loved Poems of the American People,* ed. H. Fellerman (New York: Doubleday, 1936), p. 581.

FIVE: SYNCHRONICITY

Page 87, *"She [dreamt]...someone had given"*: Carl Jung, *Synchronicity: An Acausal Connecting Principle* (New York: Pantheon, 1960), p. 109.

SIX: ANIMALS WHO SERVE

Page 107, *"Tiger's temperament is as soft"*: Jessie Walker quoted in Terri Crisp and Cynthia Hurn, *No Buddy Left Behind: Bringing U.S. Troops' Dogs and Cats Safely Home from the Combat Zone* (Guilford, CT: Lyons Press, 2011), p. 110.

Page 107, *Today Sherlock is wearing*: See a video of Sherlock: *KLM Lost and Found Service*, KLM on YouTube, posted on September 23, 2014, www.youtube.com/watch?v =NK-T_t166TY.

Page 108, *"When your dog is looking"*: "The Smartest Dog in the World," *60 Minutes*, CBS News, October 5, 2014, www.cbsnews.com/news/the-smartest-dog-in-the-world/.

SEVEN: PAW PROFESSORS

Page 131, *"The great pleasure of a dog"*: Samuel Butler, *The Notebooks of Samuel Butler*, ed. H. F. Jones (London: Fifield, 1912), p. 220.

EIGHT: SOMETIMES THEY JUST KNOW

Page 147, *"If a dog will not come to you"*: Woodrow Wilson, *Address to Congress, Analyzing German and Austrian Peace Utterances*, February 11, 1918, available at World War I Document Archive, www.gwpda.org/1918/wilpeace.html.

NINE: MIRACLE HEALERS

Page 161, *"Without your wound, where would your power be?"*: Thornton Wilder, *The Angel That Troubled the Waters and Other Plays* (New York: Coward-McCann, 1928), p. 149.

Page 175, *"I got a zoo, I got a menagerie"*: Carl Sandburg, "Wilderness," in *Cornhuskers* (Whitefish, MT: Kessinger, 2004), p. 33.

TEN: THE PSYCHIC CONNECTION

Page 179, *"I don't know what you should do"*: Amelia Kinkade, *The Language of Miracles: A Celebrated Psychic Teaches You to Talk to Animals* (Novato, CA: New World Library, 2006), p. 299.

Page 186, *"Captain Harris"*: Condensed from ibid.

Page 189, *"Captain Harris is one of the Royal procession Horses"*: Captain Harris's name has been changed.

ELEVEN: TALK TO THE ANIMALS

Page 197, *"Being a therapist for animals is no different"*: Amelia Kinkade, *The Language of Miracles: A Celebrated Psychic Teaches You to Talk to Animals* (Novato, CA: New World Library, 2006), p. 209.

TWELVE: ANIMALS AND DREAMS

Page 215, *"Your dreams, what you hope for"*: Barbara Kingsolver, *Animal Dreams* (New York: HarperCollins, 2013), p. 136.

Page 217, *"There is a land of the living"*: Thornton Wilder, *The Bridge of San Luis Rey and Other Novels* (New York: Library of America, 2009), p. 192.

Thirteen: Grief and Forgiveness

Page 233, *"In grief we can be more connected to loss"*: Elisabeth Kübler-Ross and David Kessler, *On Grief and Grieving* (New York: Scribner, 2014), p. 93.

Fourteen: Life Goes On

Page 255, *"A little while, and my longing"*: Kahlil Gibran, *The Prophet* (London: William Heinemann, 1997), p. 113.

Page 256, *"The earth circled away"*: William Saroyan, "The Daring Young Man on the Flying Trapeze," in *The Daring Young Man on the Flying Trapeze and Other Stories* (New York: New Directions, 1941), p. 25.

Page 275, *"Love is immortal"*: William Saroyan, *The Human Comedy* (New York: Harcourt Brace, 1943), p. 275.

Story Contributors

(listed alphabetically)

Floss Azzariti, Westborough, Massachusetts

C. M. Barrett, Ruby, New York
Author of *Big Dragons Don't Cry*,
www.adragonsguide.com

Jeanna Barrett, Glastonbury, England

Barb Bland, Oak Harbor, Washington
Author of *Running Free*, www.runningfreethebook.com

Audrey B. Carlson, Newington, Connecticut
Founder of Elizabeth Anne Carlson Performing Arts
Foundation, www.elizabethannecarlsonscholarship.com
/about.html

Ann Chessman, Lake Stevens, Washington

Darlene Cloud, Livermore, California

Janet Elizabeth Colli, PhD, Seattle, Washington
Author of *The Dark Face of Heaven: True Stories of Transcendence through Trauma*, www.sacredencounters.com

Terri Crisp, Somerset, California
Coauthor of *No Buddy Left Behind: Bringing U.S. Troops' Dogs and Cats Safely Home from the Combat Zone*, with
Cynthia J. Hurn

Dr. Scott Fried, Blue Bell, Pennsylvania

Author of *A Surgeon's Self-Hypnosis Healing Solution;* founder of Doctor in the House, www.docinthehouse.com

Leslie Green, St. Petersburg, Florida

R. Ira Harris, Sacramento, California

Author of *Island of the White Rose,* www.islandofthe whiterose.com

Barbara J. Hollace, Spokane Valley, Washington

Writer, editor, www.barbarahollace.com

Cindy Hurn, Norfolk, England

Hypnotherapist, personal development and spiritual transformation mentor, www.cindyhurn.com

Cynthia J. Hurn, Somerset, England

Coauthor of *The Art of Healing* (with Bernie Siegel) and *No Buddy Left Behind* (with Terri Crisp), www.brokenpenwriter.wordpress.com

Nick Hurn, Norfolk, England

Andrea Hurst, Coupeville, Washington

Coauthor of *Lazy Dog's Guide to Enlightenment* and author of *The Guestbook,* www.andreahurst.com and www.andreahurst-author.com

Michele Jane, Shropshire, England

Animal intuitive, founder of Animal Kin, www.michelejane.com

Steve J'mo, Cornwall, England

Author of *The True Story of Bilbo: The Surf Lifeguard Dog*

Geoff Johnson, Somerset, England

Homeopathic veterinarian, www.vethomeopath.co.uk

Lyn Kiernan, Freeland, Washington

Amelia Kinkade, Los Angeles, California

Author of *The Language of Miracles: A Celebrated Psychic Teaches You to Talk to Animals* and *Straight from the Horse's Mouth,* www.ameliakinkade.com

Mark S. Kuhar, Medina, Ohio

Veronica Leigh, Terre Haute, Indiana
Blogger, www.veronicaleigh.blogspot.com

Ali Le-Mar, Somerset, England

Carolyn Siegel McGaha, Woodbridge, Connecticut

Martha Pound Miller, Portland, Oregon

Alyson B. Miller-Greenfield, Lafayette, Colorado
Cofounder of Venture Growth, www.venturegrowth.com

Carolyn Monachelli, Stratford, Connecticut

Lisa L. Owens, Issaquah, Washington
Author of *Space Neighbors*, lisa@llowens.com

Jenny Pavlovic, Afton, Minnesota
Author of *The "Not without My Dog" Resource & Record Book* and *8 State Hurricane Kate*, www.8statekate.net

Terry Persun, Port Townsend, Washington
Author of *Doublesight*, www.terrypersun.com

Janice Peters, Morro Bay, California

Kay Pfaltz, Charlottesville, Virginia
Author of *Flash's Song* and *Lauren's Story*, www.kaypfaltz.com

Janet Pfeiffer, Oak Ridge, New Jersey
Author of *The Secret Side of Anger*, www.pfeifferpower seminars.com

Sandra Pollard, Whidbey Island, Washington
Author of *Puget Sound Whales for Sale: The Fight to End Orca Hunting*, www.sandrapollard.com

Cari L. Sadler, Tampa, Florida

Kathy Sdao, Tacoma, Washington
Author of *Plenty in Life Is Free: Reflections on Dogs, Training, and Finding Grace*, founder of Bright Spot Dog Training, www.kathysdao.com

Doreen Semmens, Ladysmith, B.C., Canada

Kristen Weindorf Short, Norway, Maine
    Singer, songwriter, www.kshort.com
Charlie Siegel, Granby, Connecticut
    Photography by SC, www.etsy.com/shop/photobysc
Rita Celone Umile, Cheshire, Connecticut
Ruth Vanden Bosch, Holland, Michigan
Carmen Van Etten, Germany
Dorie Walden, Hamden, Connecticut
Sandy Weinberg, Bethel, Connecticut
Gloria Wendroff, Fairfield, Iowa
    Author of *I Hear God Speak: The Story of Heaven Letters,*
    www.heavenletters.org
Rowena Williamson, Coupeville, Washington
    Author of *MacGregor's Bargain,* www.culloden-books.com
Chelsea Wolf, New York
    Singer, songwriter, *Songs from the Underground,*
    www.chelseawolf.com
Sonia S. Wolshin, Marina del Rey, California

About Bernie S. Siegel

Bernie S. Siegel, MD, is a well-known proponent of integrative and holistic approaches to healing that heal not just the body but also the mind and soul. Bernie, as his friends and patients call him, attended Colgate University and studied medicine at Cornell University Medical College. His surgical training took place at Yale–New Haven Hospital, West Haven Veterans Hospital, and the Children's Hospital of Pittsburgh. In 1978 Bernie pioneered a new approach to group and individual cancer therapy called Exceptional Cancer Patients (ECaP), which utilized patients' drawings, dreams, and feelings, and he broke new ground in facilitating important patient lifestyle changes and engaging the patient in the healing process.

Bernie retired from his general and pediatric surgical practice in 1989. Always a strong advocate for his patients, he has since dedicated himself to humanizing the medical establishment's approach to patients and empowering patients to play a vital role in the process of self-induced healing to achieve their greatest potential. He continues to run support groups and is an active speaker, traveling around the world to address patient and caregiver groups. As the author of several books — including *Love, Medicine & Miracles*; *Peace, Love & Healing*; *How to Live between Office Visits*; *365 Prescriptions for the Soul*; *Faith, Hope & Healing*; and *A Book of Miracles* — Bernie has been at the forefront of the spiritual and medical ethics issues of our day. He has been named one of the top twenty Spiritually Influential Living People by *Watkins' Mind Body Spirit* magazine (London). Bernie and his wife (and occasional coauthor), Bobbie, live in a suburb of New Haven, Connecticut. They have five children, eight grandchildren, four cats, two dogs, and much love. Visit his website at www.berniesiegelmd.com.

About Cynthia J. Hurn

Freelance writer and editor Cynthia J. Hurn is coauthor of the nonfiction books *No Buddy Left Behind: Bringing U.S. Troops' Dogs and Cats Safely Home from the Combat Zone; The Art of Healing*; and *Not My Secret to Keep: A Memoir of Healing from Childhood Sexual Abuse*. Her studies in psychology, counseling, and creative writing, plus volunteer work with animals and rescued wild birds, bring a unique mixture of science, heart, and soul to her writing. In 2014 Cynthia founded Café Write Writer's Workshop in Somerset, England. She lives with her golden retriever at her home in Exmoor National Park.

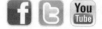